BETA AGONISTS IN THE TREATMENT OF ASTHMA

BETA AGONISTS IN THE TREATMENT OF ASTHMA

The Proceedings of a Symposium held at the Royal Society of Medicine, London, February 1992

Edited by J.F. Costello and R.D. Mann

The Parthenon Publishing Group
International Publishers in Medicine, Science & Technology

Casterton Hall, Carnforth,
Lancs, LA6 2LA, UK

One Blue Hill Plaza, Pearl River,
New York 10965, USA

Published in the UK by
The Parthenon Publishing Group Limited
Casterton Hall, Carnforth,
Lancs, LA6 2LA, UK

Published in the USA by
The Parthenon Publishing Group Inc.
One Blue Hill Plaza,
PO Box 1564, Pearl River,
New York 10965, USA

British Library Cataloguing in Publication Data
Beta Agonists in the Treatment of Asthma
I. Costello, J. F. II. Mann, R. D.
616.2

ISBN 1-85070-438-4

Library of Congress Cataloging-in-Publication Data
Beta agonists in the treatment of asthma/edited by J. F. Costello and R. D. Mann.
p. cm.
Includes bibliographical references and index.
ISBN 1-85070-438-4 :
1. Adrenergic beta agonists—Congresses. 2. Asthma—Chemotherapy—Congresses. I. Costello, J. F. (John Francis). 1944–
II. Mann, Ronald D. (Ronald David), 1928–
[DNLM: 1. Adrenergic Beta Receptor Agonists—pharmacology—congresses. 2. Adrenergic Beta Receptor Agonists—therapeutic use—congresses. 3. Asthma—drug therapy—congresses. WF 553 BN5625]
RC591.B46 061 1992
616.2′38′061—dc20
DNLM/DLC 92-49662
for Library of Congress CIP

First published 1992

Typeset by AMA Graphics Ltd., Preston, Lancashire
Printed and bound in Great Britain by
The Cromwell Press Limited, Broughton Gifford, Melksham, Wiltshire

Contents

List of principal contributors

N. C. Barnes
London Chest Hospital
Bonner Road
London E2 9JX
UK

P. J. Barnes
Department of Thoracic Medicine
National Heart and Lung Institute
Dovehouse Street
London SW3 6LY
UK

R. Beasley
Department of Medicine
Wellington School of Medicine
PO Box 7343
Wellington South
New Zealand

J. F. Costello
Department of Thoracic Medicine
King's College School of Medicine and Dentistry
Bessemer Road
London SE5 9PJ
UK

R. W. Fuller
Department of Respiratory Medicine
Glaxo Group Research Ltd
Greenford Road
Greenford
Middlesex UB6 0HE
UK

S. T. Holgate
Immunopharmacology
Southampton General Hospital
Tremona Road
Southampton SO9 4XY
UK

P. H. Howarth
Faculty of Medicine
Southampton General Hospital
Tremona Road
Southampton SO9 4XY
UK

M. Johnson
Peripheral Pharmacology
Glaxo Group Research Ltd
Ware
Hertfordshire SG12 0DP
UK

R. D. Mann
The Royal Society of Medicine
1 Wimpole Street
London W1M 8AE
UK

J. Morley
Preclinical Pharmacology
Sandoz Pharma Ltd
CH-4002 Basel
Switzerland

C. P. Page
Department of Pharmacology
King's College London
Manresa Road
London SW3 6LX
UK

M. R. Sears
McMaster University/St Joseph's Hospital
Firestone Regional Chest & Allergy Unit
50 Charlton Avenue East
Hamilton
Ontario L8N 4A6
Canada

W. Spitzer
Department of Epidemiology and Biostatistics,
McGill University
Purvis Hall
1020 Pine Avenue West
Montreal
Quebec
Canada H3A 1B2

A. E. Tattersfield
Respiratory Medicine Unit
City Hospital
Hucknall Road
Nottingham NG5 1PB
UK

Introduction

J. F. Costello

The Respiratory Section of the Royal Society of Medicine was inaugurated in October, 1991; this meeting was, therefore, only the second time that the Section had met – and the interest in both the Section and topic chosen for this meeting was gratifying, as reflected by a capacity attendance. The audience included several distinguished invited guests – Professor Sir James Black (Nobel Laureate), Professor Peter Burney (respiratory epidemiologist) and Professor W. Asscher (Chairman, Committee on Safety of Medicines).

The title of the symposium was 'β-Agonists in Asthma: State of the Art'. The first session (chaired by Professor S. T. Holgate) focused on basic mechanisms and the second session (chaired by the President of the Section) concentrated on the epidemiological and clinical aspects.

The use of β-agonists for the treatment of asthma has steadily increased throughout the world, and in the UK in particular[1]. The British Thoracic Society[2] guidelines recommend their use, as do the guidelines of the United States National Institutions of Health[3]. Both sets of guidelines stress, however, that inhaled 'anti-inflammatory' therapy, such as the use of inhaled corticosteroids, should be the mainstay of regular treatment, with β-agonists used on an as-required basis. The recent introduction of longer acting β-agonists, such as salmeterol and formoterol, and claims for an inherent 'anti-inflammatory' action of salmeterol in particular, have generated much discussion about where precisely these drugs fit into the therapeutic regimen clinicians might follow.

The debate is, however, not just about efficacy, but also about safety. Since the late 1960s there has been concern about the potential toxicity of these drugs[4,5] and these worries have been fuelled by more recent reports (several by authors who are contributors to this symposium) about new increases in asthma deaths in several countries; some of these reports appeared to implicate the regular use of β-agonist inhalers as a possible causative factor. Potential mechanisms suggested for dangerous adverse effects of β-agonists include: increased bronchial hyper-responsiveness; worsening of airway inflammation by allowing access to a greater antigen load; interference with possible beneficial actions of mast cells; and the generation of cardiac dysrhythmias and hypokalaemia. Clinically it was suggested that patients come to rely too much on the immediate bronchodilator effects of their β-agonists and, as a consequence, tend to neglect their concurrent 'anti-inflammatory' therapies.

A recent statement from the Committee on Safety of Medicines[6] suggests that the causal relationship between β-agonist use and asthma mortality is not proven. However, these arguments are countered by assertions that the epidemiological data are insufficient and relate largely to mortality, and therefore to relatively small numbers of patients, and not to morbidity which is, numerically at least, a much more formidable problem. Furthermore, there is considerable speculation as to whether any deleterious effects are due to β-agonists as a class of drugs or to specific agents.

The outcome of the debate has clear and important implications for clinical practice, and therefore for patients. It was the aim of this symposium to present a balanced discussion of the issues, with contributions to the understanding of β-receptor function and human and animal pharmacology of β-agonists, their possible effects on the pathophysiological mechanisms of asthma, the epidemiological concerns about their use and, finally, the clinical utility of β-agonists in general and the longer acting agents in particular.

We are grateful to the following pharmaceutical companies for substantial grants which made this symposium possible: Astra Pharmaceuticals, Boehringer Ingelheim, Napp Laboratories, Ciba-Geigy Pharmaceuticals. We are also grateful to Miss Judy Cook and her staff at the Royal Society of Medicine for organizing this meeting; to Dr Mary Firth for transcribing the discussion; and to Parthenon Publishing for this publication.

REFERENCES

1. Costello, J. (1991). Asthma – a United Kingdom view; treatment and its implications. *Ann. N. Y. Acad. Sci.*, **629**, 7–14
2. British Thoracic Society, Research Unit of the Royal College of Physicians of London, Kings Fund Centre, National Asthma Campaign (1990). Guidelines for management of asthma in adults. 1. Chronic persistent asthma. *Br. Med. J.*, **301**, 797–800

3. National Asthma Education Programme. (1991). *Expert Panel Report.* Publication No. 91. 3042. (Bethesda, MD: National Heart, Lung, and Blood Institute, National Institutes of Health)
4. Speizer, F. E., Doll, R. and Heap, P. (1968). Observations on recent increase in mortality from asthma. *Br. Med. J.*, **1**, 335–9
5. Inman, W. H. W. and Adelstein, A. M. (1969). Rise and fall of asthma mortality in England and Wales in relation to the use of pressurized aerosols. *Lancet*, **2**, 279–85
6. Committee on Safety of Medicines Working Party (1992). *Beta-agonist use in asthma: report from the CSM Working Party.* CSM Current Problems No. 33. February, 1992

1

Molecular pharmacology of β-adrenoceptors

P. J. Barnes

INTRODUCTION

Important advances in our understanding of the molecular mechanisms of β-adrenoceptors have recently been made, which have implications for elucidating β-adrenoceptor function in airway disease and the mechanisms of action of β-adrenoceptor agonists. At least three β-adrenoceptors are now recognized. β_1-Receptors, which are preferentially activated by noradrenaline, are physiologically regulated by sympathetic nerves; β_2-receptors, preferentially regulated by circulating adrenaline; β_3-receptors or 'atypical' β-receptors are linked to lipolysis. β_2-Receptors predominate in the lung and mediate most of the effects of β-agonists on airway function.

β-ADRENOCEPTOR STRUCTURE

Three β-adrenoceptors have now been cloned[1–4], all of which have the characteristic structure associated with G-protein-coupled receptors of seven hydrophobic stretches of 20–25 amino acids which cross the cell membrane. The intervening hydrophilic sections are exposed alternately intracellularly and extracellularly with the amino (N)-terminal exposed to the outside and the carboxy (C)-terminal within the cytoplasm (Figure 1). The molecular weight of the cloned receptors predicted from the complementary DNA (cDNA) sequence is less than the molecular mass of the wild receptors when assessed by sodium dodecyl sulphate–polyacrylamide gel electrophoresis. This discrepancy is due to glycosylation of the native receptor. For example, β_2-receptors contain two sites for glycosylation on asparagine (Asn/N) residues near the amino-terminal, and it is estimated that *N*-glycosylation accounts for 25–30% of the molecular mass of the

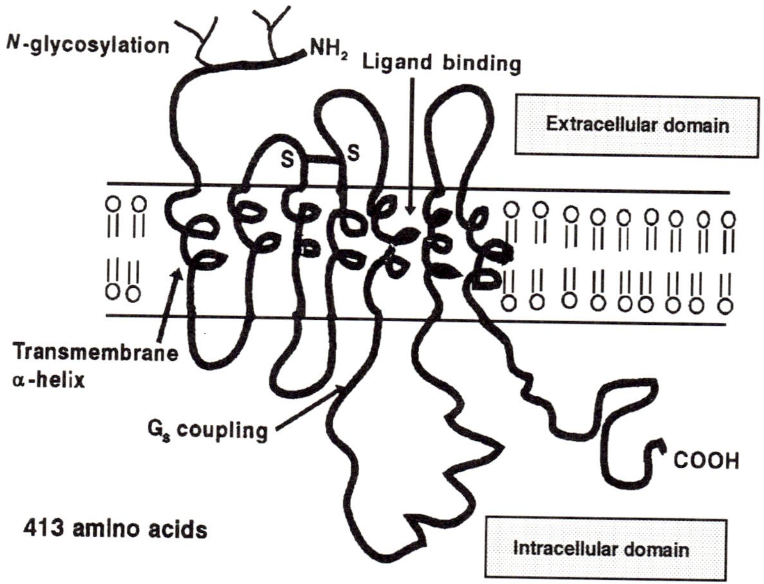

Figure 1 Structure of the human β_2-adrenoceptor: the amino acid chain has seven membrane-spanning hydrophobic regions in the form of α-helices. There is a disulphide bridge between two extracellular loops which stabilizes the three-dimensional shape of the receptor. There are two glycosylation sites. The ligand binding site is deep within the membrane between segments III and V. The third intracellular loop is important for interaction with G_S

native receptor. The functional significance of glycosylation is not yet clear; it does not affect receptor affinity for ligand binding or coupling to G-proteins but may be important for the trafficking of the receptor through the cell during down-regulation, or for keeping the receptor correctly oriented in the lipid bilayer.

The three β-receptors so far identified have distinctly different sequences. The human β_1-receptor has only 54% homology with the human β_2-receptor[5]. An atypical β-receptor, which does not clearly fit into the β_1- or β_2-receptor subtypes, has been suspected in adipose tissue and recently a 'β_3'-receptor has been identified, cloned, sequenced and expressed[4]. The β_3-receptor is clearly different from either β_1- or β_2-receptors (about 50% amino acid sequence homology). β_3-receptors appear to be important in regulation of metabolic rate and have not yet been detected in lung homogenates.

Once the cDNA sequence for receptors is known it is possible to substitute single nucleotide bases at different positions in the sequence and thus produce a mutant receptor with predetermined alterations in its amino acid sequence. This is carried out by substituting the codon for one amino acid with that for another in a synthetic oligonucleotide, and creating a mutant gene which, when expressed, produces a receptor with minor specific changes. The technique of site-directed mutagenesis has proved to be invaluable in elucidating receptor structure and function[6,7]. Replacement of the cysteine (Cys) residues at positions 106 and 184 in the second and third extracellular domain in the hamster lung β_2-receptor shows that they are important in maintaining the correct three-dimensional shape of the receptor in the cell membrane by the formation of a disulphide link between the two loops. Substitution of either of these Cys residues with isoleucine (Ile) impairs β-receptor ligand binding affinity[8]. Similarly, substitution of either of the adjacent Cys residues at positions 190 and 191 on the third cytoplasmic loop of the human β_2-receptor markedly reduces binding affinity and coupling to adenyl cyclase[9]. It is interesting that the Cys residues on the second and third extracellular loops are highly conserved amongst receptors. This suggests that they may be important in stabilizing their three-dimensional structure.

One of the most intriguing questions is the location of the ligand binding site and the means by which an agonist changes the receptor so that it can interact with the appropriate G-protein. The ligand binding domain of the β-receptor has been carefully characterized by selective deletion of sections of the gene encoding the hydrophilic and hydrophobic domains of the receptor protein, expressing the mutant receptor genes in mammalian cell lines, and determining the binding and functional characteristics of the mutant receptor. These elegant studies have demonstrated that regions which form junctions between the transmembrane hydrophobic segments and the extramembranous loops result in altered protein folding. Curiously, most of the extracellular portions of the receptor can be deleted without affecting binding, which implicates regions within the hydrophobic membrane portion as being critical for binding[10]. Site-directed mutagenesis of single amino acids of the β_2-receptor have indicated that substitution of neutral amino acids for aspartate (Asp) residues in the second and third transmembrane segments affect agonist binding affinity, but do not affect stimulatory G-proteins (G_S) activation. The importance of Asp residues may relate to the fact that they are believed to bind to the protonated group of catecholamines[6,7,11]. Interestingly, equivalent Asp residues are conserved in all other adrenergic receptors which all bind ligands with a charged amine group.

Site-directed mutagenesis of serine (Ser) residues, which may form a hydrogen bond with the catechol ring, suggests that Ser residues in the fifth transmembrane helix are important. These studies indicate that a ligand binding pocket may fit between the third and sixth transmembrane helices[6]. Using the fluorescent β-blocker carazolol, which binds with high affinity to the β_2-receptor, it has been possible with fluorescence spectroscopy to demonstrate in quenching experiments that the ligand binding site is buried deep (at least 1.1 nm) within the receptor[12].

The reason why β_2-receptors prefer adrenaline (which is more bulky), is not completely understood. Recent studies with chimaeric receptors, which are a combination of the sequence of β_1- and β_2-receptors, indicate that the sequences of amino acids in transmembrane helices 4 and 5 are critical and probably determine the shape of the binding pocket[13].

The intracellular loops located on the inner surface of the plasma membrane interact with G-proteins. Deletion mutagenesis studies, in which stretches of the amino acid sequence are removed, indicate that the third intracellular loop is critical for interaction between β_2-receptors and G_S[14]. This loop contains a sequence of amino acids which include charged amino acids in the form of an α-helix. A similar sequence is found in all G-protein-linked receptors and the third cytoplasmic loop is also present in muscarinic receptors[15].

The presence of β_2-receptor messenger RNA (mRNA) has been detected in human and rat lung by Northern blot analysis using radiolabelled cDNA (or cRNA) probes[16]. β_2-receptor mRNA has been localized by *in situ* hybridization and corresponds, as expected, to β-receptor binding sites. However, there are discrepancies between the relative density of mRNA and of receptors in certain cells. Thus, in airway smooth muscle there is a very high density of β-receptor mRNA, whereas the density of the β-receptors is relatively low; this suggests either that the rate of receptor synthesis is high, and there is a rapid turnover of receptors, or that the stability of mRNA is high. This may explain why it is difficult to down-regulate β-receptors in airway smooth muscle, and therefore to demonstrate tachyphylaxis to the bronchodilator action of β-agonists. By contrast, in the alveolar walls there is a low level of mRNA but a very high receptor density, which may indicate a low receptor turnover, and this would be consistent with the fact that down-regulation is readily produced in lung parenchyma.

INTRACELLULAR MECHANISMS

The intracellular mechanisms involved in mediating the effects of β-agonists are now reasonably well established. Occupation of a β-receptor by an agonist results in a conformational change which leads to the activation of G_S. This in turn activates the cell surface-associated enzyme adenyl cyclase, which results in conversion of ATP to cyclic 3′,5′AMP, the second messenger of β-receptor function. Cyclic AMP activates protein kinase A, which then phosphorylates certain key proteins in the cell leading to the characteristic cellular response. In airway smooth muscle, protein kinase A inhibits myosin light chain phosphorylation[17], and phosphoinositide hydrolysis[18] and promotes calcium/sodium ion exchange[19], thus resulting in a fall in intracellular calcium ions. These effects are observed only at relatively high concentrations of β-agonist, however. An important effect of β-agonists is the opening of membrane potassium channels. Charybdotoxin, which is a selective blocker of large conductance calcium-activated potassium channels (maxi-K channels) inhibits the bronchodilator responses to β-agonists and to other agents which elevate cyclic AMP[20]. These effects are observed at low concentrations of β-agonists in human airways *in vitro*, suggesting that this is a major mechanism of airway smooth muscle response to β-agonists[21]. Patch clamp studies have confirmed that elevation of cyclic AMP opens a maxi-K channel in airway smooth muscle cells[22].

LOCALIZATION AND FUNCTION

β-Adrenoceptors are present in high density in lung tissue and are localized to many different cell types. The predominant action of β-agonists is relaxation of airway smooth muscle, and β-receptors are localized to airway smooth muscle of the airways from the trachea to the terminal bronchioles[23]. These receptors are entirely of the β_2-receptor subtype in human airways, consistent with the absence of a functional adrenergic innervation[24].

Autoradiographic mapping studies also show that β-receptors are localized to submucosal glands and to airway epithelium[24]. This is consistent with the effects of β-agonists on airway secretions. β-Agonists selectively stimulate mucous rather than serous cells of submucosal glands, resulting in a viscous mucus secretion[25]. Autoradiographic mapping shows the localization of β-receptors to mucous rather than serous cells[26]. In human airways the majority of β-receptors are of the β_2 subtype, but β_1-receptors are also present consistent with adrenergic innervation of these glands. High dose β-agonists may stimulate a viscous mucus secretion which may contribute to the plugging of the airways; this is a potentially deleterious effect which has received surprisingly little attention.

β-Receptors may also influence airway blood vessels. β-Agonists cause vasodilatation, which is potentially deleterious by increasing the blood flow to leaky vessels, but β-agonists may also inhibit airway microvascular leakage. While intravenously administered β-agonists are ineffective in inhibiting plasma exudation in guinea-pigs[27], they are effective in inhibiting the leakage induced by inhaled mediators when given by the aerosol route, indicating that high local concentrations may be useful in inhibiting airway oedema[28].

β-Agonists may also modulate neurotransmission in airways. β_2-Receptors modulate cholinergic neurotransmission in human airways[29] and the release of neuropeptides from sensory nerves in rodent airways[30].

The effect of β-agonists on airway inflammation is a controversial area[31]. β-Agonists clearly inhibit the release of mediators such as histamine and leukotrienes from mast cells, and therefore can be considered to reduce acute allergic inflammation. However, there is less convincing evidence that they have effects on the cells which are believed to participate in chronic inflammation. β-Agonists have no effect on mediator release from alveolar macrophages[32], and have only a transient effect on mediator release from eosinophils[33,34]. β-Agonist effects on lymphocytes are also transient.

REGULATION OF β-RECEPTORS

Desensitization

Tachyphylaxis or desensitization occurs with most receptors when exposed to an agonist. This phenomenon has been studied in some detail with β_2-receptors and involves several processes[5,35]. In the short term, desensitization involves phosphorylation which uncouples the receptor from G_S, via the action of an enzyme called β-adrenergic receptor-specific kinase[36]. The site of this phosphorylation appears to be on the Ser/threonine (Thr) rich region of the third intracellular loop and the carboxy-terminal tail, since their replacement reduces the rate of desensitization[35,37]. Longer term mechanisms include down-regulation of surface receptor number, a process which involves internalization of the receptor and its subsequent degradation. In a cultured hamster cell line, down-regulation of β_2-receptors resulted in a rapid decline in the steady-state level of β_2-receptor mRNA[38,39]. This suggests that down-regulation is achieved in part, either by inhibiting the genetic transcription of receptors or by increasing post-transcriptional processing of the mRNA in the cell. Using actinomycin D to inhibit transcription it has been found that β_2-receptor mRNA stability is markedly reduced in these cells after exposure to β-agonists. There is some evidence that with prolonged exposure there may also be inhibition of gene transcription[40]. The various mechanisms of down-regulation have not yet been investigated in pulmonary cells.

It has proved surprisingly difficult to demonstrate tachyphylaxis of the bronchodilator effect of β-agonists in asthmatic patients, although a small effect has been observed in normal subjects[41]. This is consistent with the resistance of airway smooth muscle to down-regulation, possibly because of the high gene expression of β_2-receptors. Whether the other effects of β-agonists on airway function are equally resistant to desensitization is not certain. Recently we have demonstrated that inhaled β-agonists have a much greater protective effect against AMP-induced bronchoconstriction than against methacholine-induced constriction, suggesting that there is some extra protective effect on mast cell mediator release[42]. After 1 week of regular inhaled β-agonist (terbutaline 500 μg q.i.d.) in mild asthmatics there is no evidence for tachyphylaxis of the bronchodilator response to β-agonist, a slight reduction in protection against methacholine and a marked reduction in protective effect against AMP[42]. This may indicate tachyphylaxis of the mast cell inhibitory effect of β-agonist and provides an explanation as to why a regular β-agonist is less effective in controlling asthma symptoms than an 'on demand' β-agonist.

Steroid modulation

β-Adrenoceptors are also influenced by corticosteroids. Thus, rat pulmonary β-receptors are increased in density by pretreatment with corticosteroids[43] and corticosteroids increase the expression of β-receptors in rabbit fetal lung[44]. Steroids also prevent the desensitization and down-regulation of β-receptors on human leukocytes[45]. Corticosteroids increase the steady-state level of β_2-receptor mRNA in cultured hamster smooth muscle cells, thus indicating that steroids may increase β-receptor density by increasing the rate of gene transcription[39,46]. The increase in mRNA occurs rapidly (within 1 h), preceding the increase in β-receptors, and then declines to a steady-state level about twice that found under normal conditions. Similarly steroids increase the gene expression of β_2-receptor in human lung and in cultured airway smooth muscle cells[47]. The cloned β-receptor gene contains three potential glucocorticoid responsive elements[6].

Asthma

Whether β-receptor function in asthma is abnormal is still not resolved. There is certainly no evidence for impaired β-receptor function as a fundamental abnormality of asthma. Airway relaxation in response to β-agonists is reduced in airways obtained from patients with fatal asthma[48,49]. However, autoradiographic studies show no evidence for a reduction in β-receptor binding in airway smooth muscle[50,51], suggesting that there may be uncoupling of β-receptors rather than down-regulation. Indeed in the airways of six asthmatics who died of asthma there was a consistent increase in β-receptor density in airway smooth muscle compared with non-asthmatic controls[51], possibly as a result of increased gene transcription due to the uncoupling of β-receptors and resulting from a fall in intracellular cyclic AMP concentration. The mechanism of β-receptor uncoupling in severe asthma is uncertain, but may result from protein kinase C activation as a result of inflammatory mediator exposure.

REFERENCES

1. Frielle, T., Collins, S., Daniel, K. W., Capron, M. G., Lefkowitz, R. J. and Kobilka, B. K. (1987). Cloning of the cDNA for the β_1-adrenergic receptor. *Proc. Natl. Acad. Sci. USA*, **84**, 7920–4
2. Dixon, R. A. F., Kobilka, B. K., Strader, C. and Benovic, J. L. (1986). Cloning of the gene and cDNA for mammalian β-adrenergic receptor and homology with rhodopsin. *Nature (London)*, **321**, 75–9
3. Chung, F.-Z., Lentes, K.-U., Gocayne, J., Fitzgerald, M., Robinson, D., Kerlavage, A. R., Fraser, C. M. and Venter, J. C. (1987). Cloning and sequence analysis of the human brain β-adrenergic receptor. *FEBS Lett.*, **211**, 200–6
4. Emorine, L. J., Marullo, S., Briend-Sutren, M.-M., Patey, S., Tate, K., Delavier-Klutchkoc, C. and Strasberg, D. (1989). Molecular characterization of the human β_3-adrenergic receptor. *Science*, **245**, 1118–21
5. Lefkowitz, R. J. and Caron, M. G. (1988). Adrenergic receptors. Models for the study of receptors coupled to guanine nucleotide regulatory proteins. *J. Biol. Chem.*, **263**, 4993–6
6. Strader, C. D., Sigal, I. S. and Dixon, R. A. F. (1989). Structural basis of β-adrenergic receptor function. *FASEB J.*, **3**, 1825–32
7. Fraser, C. M. (1989). Site-directed mutagenesis of β-adrenergic receptors. *J. Biol. Chem.*, **264**, 9266–70
8. Strader, C. D., Sigal, I. S., Candelore, M. R., Rands, E., Hill, W. S. and Dixon, R. A. F. (1988). Conserved aspartic acid residues 79 and 113 of the β-adrenergic receptor have different roles in receptor function. *J. Biol. Chem.*, **263**, 10267–71
9. Fraser, C. M., Chung, F.-Z., Wang, C.-D. and Venter, J. C. (1988). Site-directed mutagenesis of human β-adrenergic receptors: substitution of aspartic acid-130 by asparagine produces a receptor with high-affinity agonist binding that is uncoupled for adenylate cyclase. *Proc. Natl. Acad. Sci. USA*, **85**, 5478–82
10. Dixon, R. A. F., Sigal, I. S., Rands, E., Register, R. B., Candelore, M. R., Blake, A. D. and Strader, C. D. (1987). Ligand binding to the β-adrenergic receptor involves its rhodopsin-like core. *Nature (London)*, **326**, 73–7

11. Chung, F.-Z., Wang, C.-D., Potter, P. C., Venter, J. C. and Fraser, C. M. (1988). Site-directed mutagenesis and continuous expression of human β-adrenergic receptors. *J. Biol. Chem.*, **263**, 4052–5
12. Tota, M. R. and Strader, C. D. (1990). Characterization of the binding domain of the β-adrenergic receptor with the fluorescent antagonist carazolol. *J. Biol. Chem.*, **265**, 16891–7
13. Kobilka, B. K., Kobilka, T. S., Daniel, K., Regan, J. W., Caron, M. G. and Lefkowitz, R. J. (1988). Chimeric α_2- and β_2-adrenergic receptors: delineation of domains involved in effector coupling and ligand specificity. *Science*, **240**, 1310–16
14. O'Dowd, B. F., Hnatowich, M., Regan, J. W., Leader, W. M., Caron, M. G. and Lefkowitz, R. J. (1988). Site-directed mutagenesis of the cytoplasmic domains of the human β_2-adrenergic receptor. *J. Biol. Chem.*, **263**, 15985–92
15. Kurtenbach, E., Curtis, C. A. M., Pedder, E. K., Aiken, A., Harris, A. C. M. and Hulme, E. C. (1990). Muscarinic acetylcholine receptors. *J. Biol. Chem.*, **265**, 13702–8
16. Hamid, Q. A., Mak, J. C., Sheppard, M. N., Corrin, B., Venter, J. C. and Barnes, P. J. (1991). Localization of β_2-adrenoceptor messenger RNA in human and rat lung using *in situ* hybridization: correlation with receptor autoradiography. *Eur. J. Pharmacol. (Mol. Pharmacol.)*, **206**, 133–8
17. Gerthoffer, U. T. (1986). Calcium dependence of myosin phosphorylation and airway smooth muscle contraction and relaxation. *Am. J. Physiol.*, **250**, C597–604
18. Hall, I. P. and Hill, S. J. (1988). Beta$_2$-adrenoceptor stimulation inhibits histamine-stimulated inositol phospholipid hydrolysis in bovine tracheal smooth muscle. *Br. J. Pharmacol.*, **95**, 1204–12
19. Twort, C. A. C. and van Breemen, C. (1989). Human airway smooth muscle in cell culture: control of the intracellular calcium store. *Pulm. Pharmacol.*, **2**, 45–53
20. Jones, T. R., Charette, L., Garcia, M. L. and Kaczorowski, G. J. (1990). Selective inhibition of relaxation of guinea-pig trachea by charybdotoxin, a potent Ca^{++}-activated K^+ channel inhibitor. *J. Pharmacol. Exp. Ther.*, **225**, 697–706
21. Miura, M., Belvisi, M. G., Stretton, C. D., Yacoub, M. H. and Barnes, P. J. (1992). Role of potassium channels in bronchodilator responses in human airways. *Am. Rev. Respir. Dis.*, in press

22. Kume, H., Takai, A., Tokuno, H. and Tomita, T. (1989). Regulation of Ca^{2+}-dependent K^+ channel activity in tracheal myocytes by phosphorylation. *Nature (London)*, **341**, 152–4
23. Carstairs, J R., Nimmo, A. J. and Barnes, P. J. (1984). Autoradiographic localisation of β-adrenoceptors in human lung. *Eur. J. Pharmacol.*, **103**, 189–90
24. Carstairs, J. R., Nimmo, A. J. and Barnes, P. J. (1985). Autoradiographic visualization of β-adrenoceptor subtypes in human lung. *Am. Rev. Respir. Dis.*, **1332**, 541–7
25. Ueki, I., German, V. and Nadel, J. (1980). Micropipette measurement of airway submucosal gland secretion: autonomic effects. *Am. Rev. Respir. Dis.*, **121**, 351–7
26. Barnes, P. J. and Basbaum, C. B. (1983). Mapping of adrenergic receptors in the trachea by autoradiography. *Exp. Lung Res.*, **5**, 183–92
27. Boschetto, P., Roberts, N. M., Rogers, D. F. and Barnes, P. J. (1989). The effect of antiasthma drugs on microvascular leak in guinea pig airways. *Am. Rev. Respir. Dis.*, **139**, 416–21
28. Tokuyama, K., Lötvall, J. Q., Löfdahl, C.-G., Barnes, P. J. and Chung, K. F. (1991). Inhaled formoterol inhibits histamine induced airflow obstruction and airway microvascular leakage. *Eur. J. Pharmacol.*, **193**, 35–40
29. Rhoden, K. J. and Barnes, P. J. (1988). Inhibition of cholinergic neurotransmission in human airways by β_2-adrenoceptors. *J. Appl. Physiol.*, **65**, 700–5
30. Verleden, G. M., Belvisi, M. G., Rabe, K. F., Miura, M. and Barnes, P. J. (1992). β_2-Adrenoceptors inhibit NANC neural bronchoconstrictor responses *in vitro*. *J. Appl. Physiol.*, in press
31. Barnes, P. J. and Chung, K. F. (1992). Questions about inhaled β_2-agonists in asthma. *Trends Pharmacol. Sci.*, **13**, 20–3
32. Fuller, R. W., O'Malley, G., Baker, A. J. and MacDermot, J. (1988). Human alveolar macrophage activation: inhibition by forskolin but not β-adrenoceptor stimulation or phosphodiesterase inhibition. *Pulm. Pharmacol.*, **1**, 101–6
33. Yukawa, T., Ukena, D., Chanez, P., Dent, G., Chung, K. F. and Barnes, P. J. (1990). Beta-adrenergic receptors on eosinophils: binding and functional studies. *Am. Rev. Respir. Dis.*, **141**, 1446–552
34. Rabe, K. F., Giembycz, M., Dent, G., Evans, P. M. and Barnes, P. J. (1992). β_2-Adrenoceptor agonists and respiratory burst activity in guinea pig peritoneal eosinophils. *Br. J. Pharmacol.*, in press
35. Bouvier, M., Collins, S., O'Dowd, B. F., Campbell, P. T., DeBlasi, A., Kabilka, B. K., MacGregor, C., Irons, G. P., Caron, M. G. and Lefkowitz,

R. J. (1989). Two distinct pathways for cAMP-mediated down-regulation of the β_2-adrenergic receptor. *J. Biol. Chem.*, **264**, 16786–92

36. Benovic, J. L., Strasser, R. H., Daniel, K. and Lefkowitz, R. J. (1986). Beta-adrenergic receptor kinase: identification of a novel protein kinase that phosphorylates the agonist-occupied form of the receptor. *Proc. Natl. Acad. Sci. USA*, **83**, 2797–801
37. Bouvier, M. W., Hausdorff, A., DeBlasi, A., O'Dowd, B. F., Kobilka, B. K., Caron, M. G. and Lefkowitz, R. J. (1988). Removal of phosphorylation sites from the β-adrenergic receptor delays the onset of agonist-promoted desensitization. *Nature (London)*, **333**, 370–3
38. Hadcock, J. R., Williams, D. L. and Malbon C. C. (1989). Physiological regulation at the level of mRNA: analysis of steady state levels of specific mRNAs by DNA-excess solution hybridization. *Am. J. Physiol.*, **256**, C457–65
39. Hadcock, J. R., Wang, H. Y. and Malbon, C. C. (1989). Agonist-induced destabilization of β-adrenergic receptor mRNA: attenuation of glucocorticoid-induced up-regulation of β-adrenergic receptors. *J. Biol. Chem.*, **264**, 19928–33
40. Collins, S., Caron, M. G. and Lefkowitz, R. J. (1992). From ligand binding to gene expression: new insights into the regulation of G-protein-coupled receptors. *Trends Pharmacol. Sci.*, **17**, 37–9
41. Tattersfield, A. E. (1985). Tolerance to beta-agonists. *Clin. Respir. Physiol.*, **21**, 1–5S
42. O'Connor, B. J., Aikman, S. L. and Barnes, P. J. (1992). Tachyphylaxis to terbutaline in asthma: evidence for a greater effect on airway mast cells than in airway smooth muscle. *Am. Rev. Respir. Dis.*, **145**, A392
43. Mano, K., Akbarzadeh, A. and Townley, R. G. (1979). Effect of hydrocortisone on beta-adrenergic receptors in lung membranes. *Life Sci.*, **25**, 1925–30
44. Barnes, P. J., Jacobs, M. M. and Roberts, J. M. (1984). Glucocorticoids preferably increase fetal alveolar beta-receptors: autoradiographic evidence. *Pediatr. Res.*, **18**, 1191–4
45. Davis, A. Q. and Lefkowitz, R. J. (1984). Regulation of β-adrenergic receptors by steroid hormones. *Ann. Rev. Physiol.*, **46**, 119–30
46. Collins, S., Caron, M. G. and Lefkowitz, R. J. (1988). β-Adrenergic receptors in hamster smooth muscle cells are transcriptionally regulated by glucocortoids. *J. Biol. Chem.*, **263**, 9067–70

47. Mak, J. C. W., Adcock, I. and Barnes, P. J. (1992). Dexamethasone increases β_2-adrenoceptor gene expression in human lung. *Am. Rev. Respir. Dis.*, **145**, A834
48. Goldie, R. G., Spina, D., Henry, P. J., Lulich, K. M. and Paterson, J. W. (1986). *In vitro* responsiveness of human asthmatic bronchus to carbachol, histamine, β-adrenoceptor agonists and theophylline. *Br. J. Clin. Pharmacol.*, **22**, 669–76
49. Bai, T. R. (1991). Abnormalities in airway smooth muscle in fatal asthma: a comparison between trachea and bronchus. *Am. Rev. Respir. Dis.*, **143**, 441–3
50. Spina, D., Rigby, P. J., Paterson, J. W. and Goldie, R. G. (1989). Autoradiographic localization of beta-adrenoceptors in asthmatic human lung. *Am. Rev. Respir. Dis.*, **140**, 1410–15
51. Bai, T. R., Mak, J. C. W. and Barnes, P. J. (1992). A comparison of β-adrenergic receptors and *in vitro* relaxant responses to isoproterenol in asthmatic airway smooth muscle. *Am. J. Respir. Cell. Mol. Biol.*, in press

DISCUSSION

Prof. Sir James Black (UK) The old idea about the β_2-receptors was that they were the ones which were coupled to nerves. Of course, there is some evidence, in laboratory animals at least, that the innervation of bronchial muscle is quite slight. This would mean that their mediation of the action of the release of noradrenaline would be by uptake. Is there any evidence that blocking uptake has bronchodilator activities?

Prof. P. J. Barnes That is a very interesting suggestion, but little effect has been observed when uptake blockers have been used. As far as we can see, there are no functional sympathetic nerves in human airways, and it is impossible to demonstrate sympathetic bronchodilatation. In species such as dog, where it can be demonstrated, uptake blockers have been looked at, and the responsiveness can be shifted to the left. In the context of clinical disease, though, it is probably not important: this mechanism could not operate because there are no nerves.

Dr J. D. Fitzgerald (Cheshire) Would you like to comment on the possible role of the non-adrenergic non-cholinergic system either physiologically or in asthma? There is a resurging interest in this at the present time. Does it have any relevance to what we are talking about today?

Prof. P. J. Barnes It could have some relevance. The non-adrenergic non-cholinergic system includes a bronchodilator pathway that we had always assumed was due to the release of the peptide, vasoactive intestinal polypeptide. There has been some evidence that vasoactive intestinal polypeptide immunoreactivity is reduced or at least absent in asthma. I think those studies are slightly confusing because there may be secondary breakdown of the peptide after death as a result of enzyme action. This is now known to be irrelevant anyway because the only neurotransmitter of the bronchodilator nerves in humans is nitric oxide, and there is no place for vasoactive intestinal polypeptide.

Perhaps of more relevance is the excitatory non-adrenergic non-cholinergic system which may involve release of peptides from sensory nerves. In the context of β-agonists, we have demonstrated that they have the capacity to inhibit non-adrenergic non-cholinergic nerves in airways. It is not clear what the relevance of these nerves would be in human asthmatic airways. They are known not to be important in the regulation of airway tone in normal humans, but they could be important in the regulation of secretions and local immunity. In asthmatics, though, they may become much more important. Recently, we have demonstrated a very striking increase in the transcription of a tachykinin (NK_1) receptor that mediates the inflammatory effects of tachykinins.

2

Mechanisms of action of β-adrenoceptor agonists

M. Johnson

β-agonists were developed in the early 1960s as analogues of adrenaline. The first of these, isoprenaline, was non-selective in that it did not discriminate between β_1 and β_2-subtypes of the β-adrenoceptor[1]. Although an effective bronchodilator, it was short-acting and its use was associated with extra-pulmonary side-effects. Salbutamol was the prototype selective β_2-agonist, showing a > 500-fold separation in activity at β_2- over β_1-receptors[2], and which has proven to be well tolerated and highly efficacious in controlling bronchospasm in over 20 years of clinical use. Since the introduction of salbutamol, a number of other β_2-agonists have been developed, ranging from more potent compounds, such as fenoterol[3] and procaterol[4], to those which were metabolically more stable, such as clenbuterol[5]. The major drawback with the first generation of β_2-agonists is their duration of action of 4–6 h, which limits their usefulness in controlling the symptoms of nocturnal asthma and in providing convenient maintenance therapy for the patient. This problem has been largely overcome with the identification of a new generation of long-acting β_2-agonists represented by salmeterol and formoterol (Figure 1). The rationale behind the design of salmeterol was to introduce large non-polar *N*-substituents into saligenin ethanolamines to facilitate specific binding in the cell membrane[6]. Such molecules would then be long-acting by persisting at their binding sites and repeatedly activating the β-adrenoceptor. In contrast, formoterol was developed by investigating β-agonist analogues with a high affinity for the β-adrenoceptor itself[7].

β-agonists exhibit a range of pharmacological properties. They share the ability to stimulate β_1-, β_2- and β_3-adrenoceptors, members of the family of seven transmembrane receptors[8], in a number of different cell types. Molecular biology studies have shown that the agonist binding site for

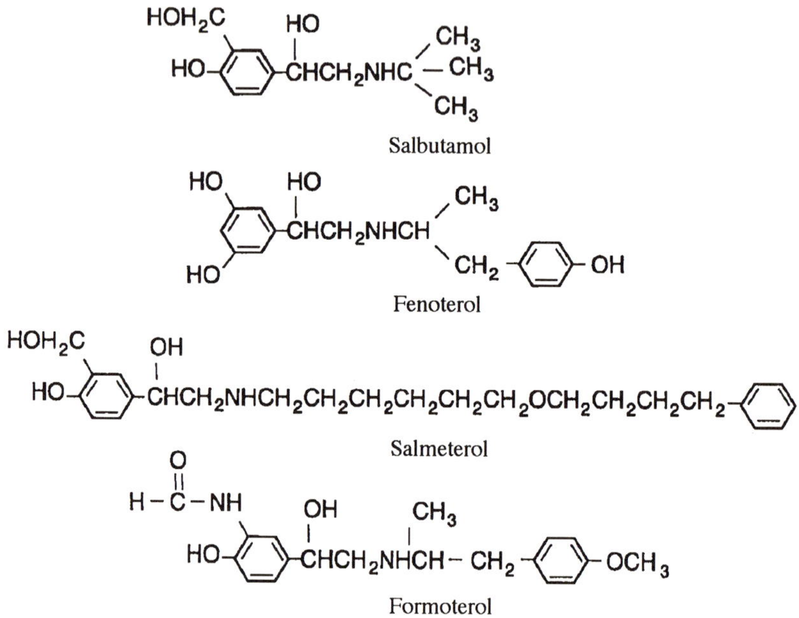

Figure 1 Structures of representative β_2-agonists

β_2-adrenoceptors is represented by serine residues, 204 and 207 in the fifth domain and aspartate residues 79 and 113 in the second and third domains respectively of the receptor protein[9]. The binding of salbutamol to the β_2-receptor is shown schematically in Figure 2a. This binding leads to activation of the receptor, dissociation of the GTP-α-subunit of the G_S-protein complex, stimulation of adenylate cyclase and the formation of cyclic AMP, which then acts as the intracellular mediator of the functional response to the β-agonist[10]. Salbutamol, and other related β-agonists, are hydrophilic molecules and appear to access the β-adrenoceptor directly. In contrast, formoterol and salmeterol are 30 and 10 000 times more lipophilic than salbutamol, respectively, and the use of high resolution physicochemical techniques[11] has shown that salmeterol approaches the active site of the β-adrenoceptor through the membrane. Salbutamol has an affinity for β_2-adrenoceptors of 2500 nmol/l compared with 200 nmol/l for isoprenaline[12]. Similar studies with salmeterol and formoterol have shown a 50-fold higher affinity, with affinity constants of 53 and 76 nmol/l respectively[13]. Furthermore, whereas isoprenaline and salbutamol readily dissociate from

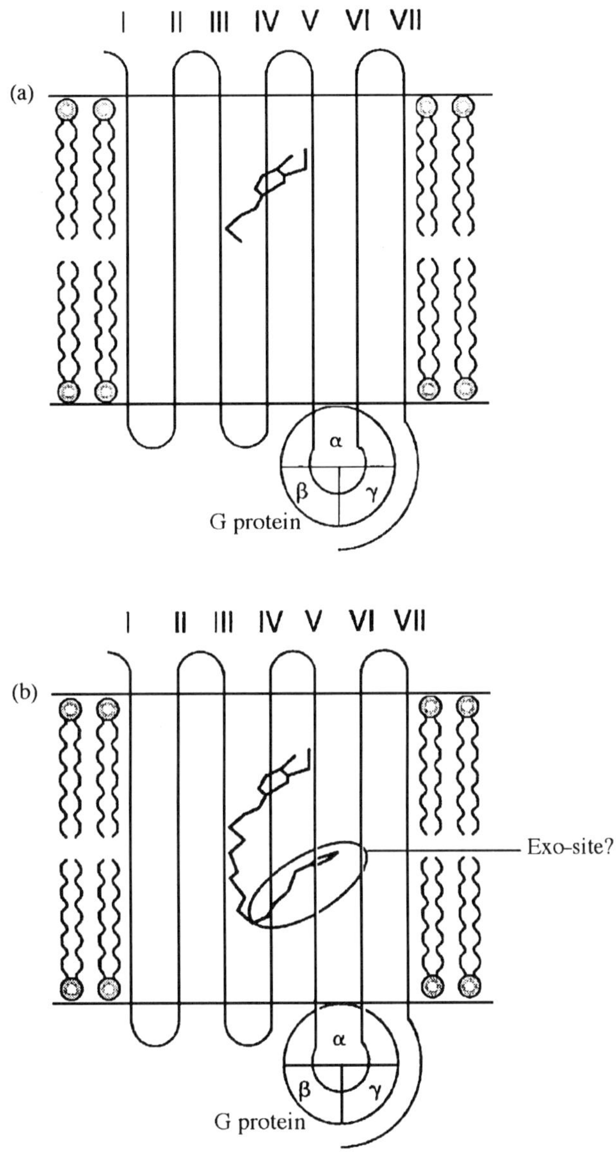

Figure 2 Predicted binding sites for (a) salbutamol and (b) salmeterol in the β_2-adrenoceptor protein

Table 1 Pharmacological effects of β-agonists

	Airways smooth muscle: β2-adrenoceptors		*Cardiac tissue: β1-adrenoceptors*		
β-agonist	*Potency*	*Efficacy (%)*	*Potency*	*Efficacy (%)*	*Selectivity ratio*
Isoprenaline	1.0	100	1.0	100	1.0
Salbutamol	0.25	86	0.0004	14	650
Fenoterol	1.0	100	0.005	100	200
Formoterol	25.0	100	0.05	100	500
Salmeterol	5.0	63	0.0001	4	50 000

their binding sites ($T_{1/2}$ = 2 min), and the dissociation of formoterol is only marginally slower ($T_{1/2}$ = 6 min), there is little evidence of dissociation of salmeterol from lung membranes for periods up to 5 h[14]. From the molecular co-ordinates of the β-receptor domains, it has been predicted that there is a preferred conformation of the salmeterol molecule in the protein (Figure 2b), whereby the active saligenin head is in an analogous position to that of adrenaline and salbutamol, and the long, flexible side-chain is located deep into a specific hydrophobic core domain of the receptor[15], which has previously been termed the 'exo-site'[16]. Binding of the side-chain to the exo-site allows the other end of the molecule to interact freely and continuously with the active site of the receptor, enabling salmeterol to be long-lasting without causing desensitization or tachyphylaxis[17]. Such a mechanism of action may explain the observation that the effects of salmeterol are rapidly and fully reversed with a β-blocking drug, but are reasserted when the β-antagonist is removed from the tissue[18]. Despite its persistent effects at the β-adrenoceptor, there is no evidence from extensive toxicological studies for accumulation of salmeterol in tissues. Similar studies have shown that formoterol does not share the mechanism of action of salmeterol[19], and the longer-lasting pharmacological effects may be explained by a combination of high affinity and efficacy, and the lipophilicity of the compound.

At β_2-adrenoceptors in airways smooth muscle *in vitro*, whereas salbutamol is four times less potent than isoprenaline, fenoterol is equipotent, and salmeterol and formoterol are more potent than isoprenaline (Table 1). Fenoterol and formoterol are full agonists at β_2-adrenoceptors, whereas salbutamol and salmeterol are partial agonists (Table 1). β-agonist molecules are usually racemic mixtures of optical isomers, there being two enantiomers

Table 2 Comparative potency of individual optical isomers of salbutamol and salmeterol

	Potency (EC_{50} (nmol/l))†
(RS)-Salbutamol	46.2
(R)-Salbutamol*	36.0
(S)-Salbutamol*	1110.0
(RS)-Salmeterol	4.8
(R)-Salmeterol	1.7
(S)-Salmeterol	80.7

*Data from reference 20; †EC_{50}, 50% effective concentration

(R and S) in salbutamol and salmeterol, and four enantiomers in fenoterol and formoterol (Figure 1). The β_2-agonist potency lies predominantly in the R-enantiomer (Table 2), but although the S-enantiomer is weaker, it still exhibits significant β_2-activity. There is no evidence of the S-isomer antagonizing the effects of the corresponding R-form[20] or of the S-enantiomer having pharmacological effects different to those of the racemate[21].

In contrast to their effects at β_2-adrenoceptors, at cardiac β_1-receptors, all of the β-agonists are less potent that isoprenaline, ranging from 20-fold for formoterol to > 10 000-fold weaker for salmeterol. Both salbutamol and salmeterol are weak partial agonists at β_1-adrenoceptors (Table 1), whereas fenoterol and formoterol have the same efficacy as isoprenaline. By comparing potency and efficacy data, it is possible to derive functional selectivity ratios for β-agonists. Fenoterol has the lowest β_2/β_1-selectivity and contrasts markedly with salmeterol which has a very high degree of β_2-selectivity (Table 1). Similarly, whereas salbutamol and salmeterol have low potency at atypical β_3-adrenoceptors[22], fenoterol and formoterol are again equivalent to isoprenaline.

In addition to differences in receptor affinity and efficacy, there are also differences in the rate of onset and duration of action of β-agonists. In isolated airways preparations, such as the guinea-pig trachea *in vitro*, all β-agonists relax the tissue either when tone is induced with a spasmogen such as prostaglandin $F_{2\alpha}$ or carbachol, or following electrical stimulation[23]. However, whereas the onset of action of isoprenaline, salbutamol and fenoterol is rapid (< 4 min), that of formoterol is somewhat delayed, and responses to salmeterol are slow to reach equilibrium under these conditions

Table 3 Time of onset and duration of action of β-agonists at β_2-adrenoceptors in guinea-pig trachea

β-*agonist*	*Onset time* (min)	*Duration of action* (min)
Isoprenaline	1.5	2.0
Salbutamol	3.2	11.0
Fenoterol	3.8	5.5
Formoterol	8.3	19.6
Salmeterol	29.0	> 720

(Table 3). In contrast, whilst isoprenaline has a short duration of action, and equipotent concentrations of salbutamol and formoterol are similar, salmeterol is long-lasting (Table 3). These differences in the duration of action of β-agonists are also apparent in the human bronchus[24] and can be extrapolated *in vivo* to bronchodilator activity in conscious animals[25] and the asthmatic patient. For example, Ullman and Svedmyr[26] confirmed that salmeterol (50 μg) has a 12-h bronchodilator action compared with 4–6 h for salbutamol (200 μg). In other studies, the duration of action of formoterol has been shown to be dose-dependent, with 6 μg inducing bronchodilatation for 8 h and higher doses being required to extend this to 12 h[27].

The pharmacological activity of β-agonists is not confined to airways smooth muscle, and they also exhibit a range of non-bronchodilator properties. For example, it has been reported previously that there are functional β_2-adrenoceptors in lung mast cells[28] and that β-agonists inhibit inflammatory mediator release[29]. Formoterol is the most potent agonist in inhibiting antigen-induced histamine release from human lung tissue *in vitro*, with a 50% inhibitory concentration (IC_{50})of 0.25 nmol/l, the rank order of potency of β-agonists being formoterol > isoprenaline > salmeterol > salbutamol. In contrast, whereas the duration of action of isoprenaline and salbutamol at mast cell β-adrenoceptors is again short (< 4 h), salmeterol has a sustained effect for up to 20 h against histamine, leukotriene C_4 and D_4 and prostaglandin D_2 release[30]. Formoterol is intermediate between salbutamol and salmeterol (Table 4). This effect of β-agonists on mast cell-derived mediator release has been demonstrated *in vivo* following antigen-challenge of sensitized subjects[31].

β-Adrenoceptors are also present in a number of other target cells, including the vascular endothelial cell. β-Agonists, by preventing contraction and maintaining the integrity of the gap junctions between the cells[32],

Table 4 Inhibition of antigen-induced histamine release from human lung by β-adrenoceptor agonists

	Potency (IC_{50} (nmol/l))	*Duration of action* (h)
Isoprenaline	1.1	2.0
Salbutamol	35.8	4.0
Formoterol	0.25	7.0
Salmeterol	3.0	> 20.0

inhibit vascular permeability and the leakage of plasma proteins from the blood into tissues. Formoterol, salbutamol and salmeterol have all been reported[33,34] to inhibit histamine-induced protein extravasation in guinea-pig airways. This effect can be shown to be β-receptor-mediated, since the inhibitory effects are reversed by pretreatment with propranolol[34]. Similarly, salmeterol given locally or systemically inhibits vascular permeability changes in the skin[35]. There are again differences in the duration of action of β-agonists at endothelial cell β-adrenoceptors, with salmeterol being effective for up to 8 h, compared with less than 2 h for salbutamol and 4 h for formoterol[34]. The bronchial epithelium also contains functional β-adrenoceptors. Salbutamol has been reported to increase the cilial beat frequency in human bronchial epithelial cells in culture[36]. This effect is modest and transient in nature. In contrast, salmeterol produces an increment in cilial beat frequency from 9.2 to 10.9 Hz, at 100-fold lower concentrations, and its effect is sustained for 15–20 h[36].

Inflammatory cells are relatively insensitive to the direct inhibitory effects of β-agonists. High concentrations ($> 10^{-6}$ mol/l) of isoprenaline, salbutamol, salmeterol and formoterol are required to inhibit eosinophil cationic protein, leukotriene B_4 and thromboxane B_2 release from human eosinophils, neutrophils[37] and alveolar macrophages[38], respectively. In contrast, *in vivo*, the long-acting β_2-agonists salmeterol and formoterol, but not salbutamol, inhibit the infiltration of inflammatory cells into the lung. Bronchodilator doses of salmeterol, given by the inhaled route, inhibit platelet activating factor or antigen-induced eosinophil accumulation in bronchoalveolar lavage fluid 24 h after challenge[39]. Similar findings have been reported for formoterol[40]. This effect is not specific to eosinophils, but equally applies to endotoxin-induced neutrophil recruitment in the rat[41], a species which does not bronchodilate to β-agonists. The inhibitory effect of salmeterol is antagonized by the β-blocker, DL-propranolol, but not by

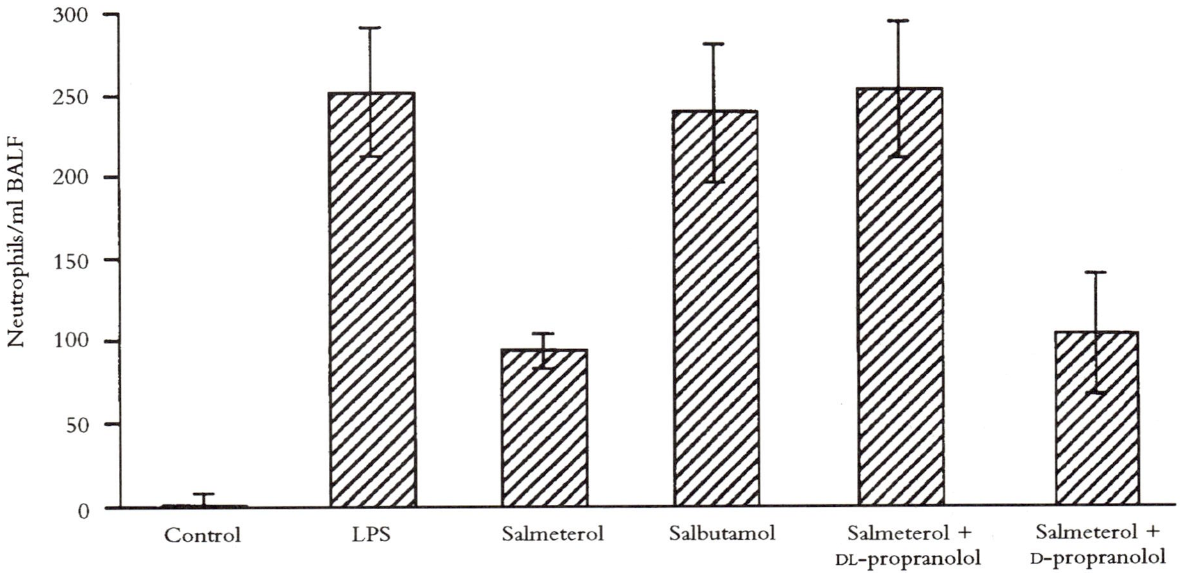

Figure 3 Effect of β_2-agonists on endotoxin-induced neutrophil accumulation in rat lung: BALF, bronchoalveolar lavage fluid; LPS, lipopolysaccharide

D-propranolol, which has no β-blocking activity (Figure 3). β-Agonists are also active against inflammatory cell recruitment in the skin, where salmeterol, by intradermal or oral administration, inhibits zymosan-induced neutrophil infiltration and granulocyte-dependent oedema[35]. This effect is not shared by the short-acting β-agonist, salbutamol. The mechanism of action of β-agonists on inflammatory cell trafficking *in vivo* is also likely to be mediated by β-adrenoceptors on endothelial cells, possibly in postcapillary venules, since it is at this level that inflammatory cells diapedese from the vascular into the tissue compartment.

There is emerging clinical evidence to support a potentially important non-bronchodilator role for β-agonists. Twentyman and colleagues[42] reported that salmeterol inhibited the late response to antigen in sensitized subjects, a response which has been associated with inflammatory changes in the airways[43] and at which conventional doses of salbutamol and terbutaline have little, if any, effect[44]. These findings have been confirmed in a second study by Fuller[45] and also reported for formoterol[46]. Both groups[42,45] have shown that salmeterol also inhibits the increase in bronchial hyperresponsiveness which follows antigen challenge for up to 48 h, a time when the drug ceases to have any bronchodilator activity. Similarly, Grönneberg and Zetterström[47] have shown that formoterol, but not terbutaline, has significant inhibitory effects on the late cutaneous reaction following anti-immunoglobulin E challenge in human skin. In addition, alveolar macrophage activation and eosinophil cationic protein levels in bronchoalveolar lavage fluid were reduced following 4 weeks of treatment of asthmatic patients with salmeterol[48]. However, a recent study by Howarth[49] failed to demonstrate an effect of salmeterol on markers of established inflammation in the lung after 6 weeks. Further work is clearly necessary before the clinical significance of the non-bronchodilator effects of the long-acting β_2-agonists in bronchial asthma can be evaluated.

In conclusion, although as a class β-adrenoceptor agonists share a number of pharmacological properties, there are marked differences in receptor affinity, efficacy, selectivity and now, duration of action between individual compounds. The mechanisms of action of β-agonists range from relaxation of airways smooth muscle and inhibition of neurotransmitter release, to effects on some of the processes of acute inflammation including suppression of inflammatory mediator release, inhibition of vascular permeability and attenuation of inflammatory cell recruitment. The latter are more apparent in the new long-acting β_2-agonists such as salmeterol, and are the result of

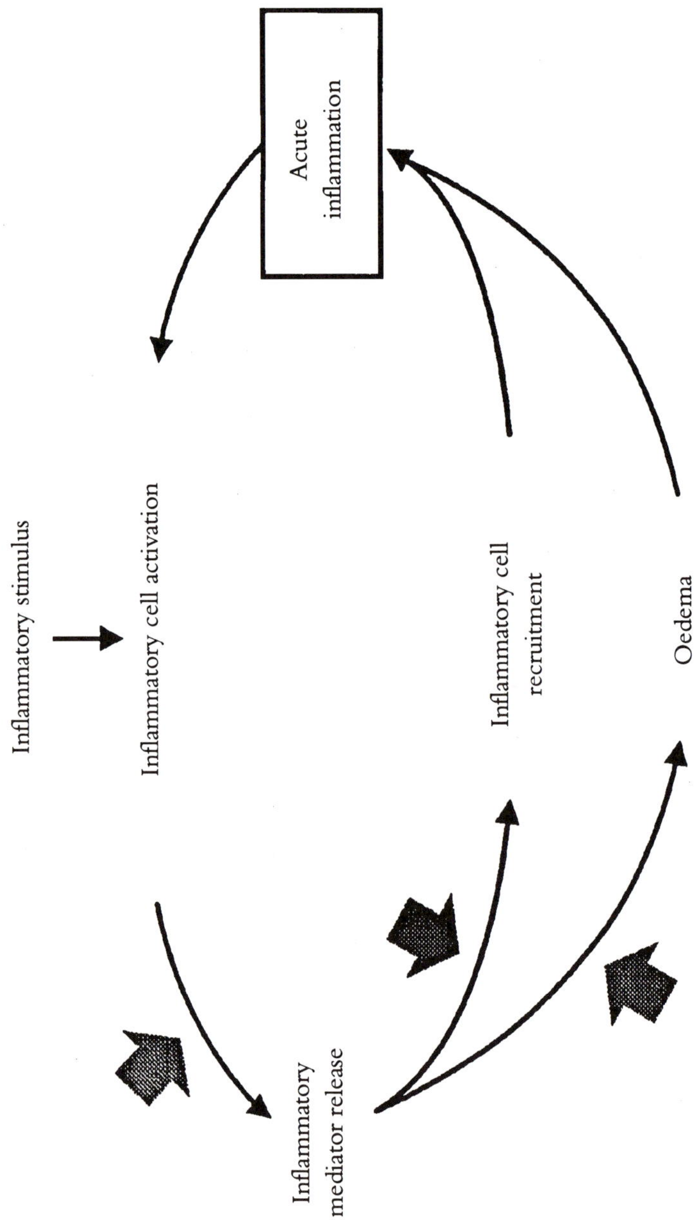

Figure 4 Functional antagonism by long-acting β_2-agonists of acute inflammatory processes

the ability of these drugs to produce potent and prolonged functional antagonism in a variety of target cells (Figure 4).

REFERENCES

1. Gay, L. N. and Long, J. W. (1949). Clinical evaluation of isopropylepinephrine in management of bronchial asthma. *J. Am. Med. Assoc.*, **139**, 452–7
2. Cullum, V. A., Farmer, J. B., Jack, D. and Levy, G. P. (1969). Salbutamol: a new, selective β-adrenoceptive receptor stimulant. *Br. J. Pharmacol.*, **35**, 141
3. Gray, B. J., Frame, M. H. and Costello, J. F. (1987). A comparative double-blind study of the bronchodilator effects and side effects of inhaled fenoterol and terbutaline administered in equipotent doses. *Br. J. Dis. Chest.*, **76**, 341–50
4. Siegel, S. C., Katz, R. M., Rachelefsky, G. S., Brandon, M. L. and Brorgen, L. A. (1985). A placebo-controlled trial of procaterol: a new, long-acting oral β_2-agonist in bronchial asthma. *J. Allergol. Immunol.*, **75**, 698–705
5. Brusasco, V., Crimi, E., Mangini, S. and Vibelli, C. (1980). A clinical trial of oral clenbuterol (NAB365) in chronic airways obstruction. *Curr. Med. Res. Opin.*, **6**, 449–55
6. Bradshaw, J., Brittain, R. T., Coleman, R. A., Jack, D., Kennedy, I., Lunts, L. H. C. and Skidmore, I. F. (1987). The design of salmeterol: a long-acting, selective β_2-adrenoceptor agonist. *Br. J. Pharmacol.*, **92**, 590P
7. Tomioka, K., Yamada, T. and Tachikama, S. (1984). Effects of formoterol (BD40A), a β-adrenoceptor stimulant, on isolated guinea-pig lung parenchymal strips and antigen-induced SRS-A release in rats. *Arch. Int. Pharmacodyn.*, **267**, 91–102
8. Kobilka, B. K., Dixon, R. A. F., Friedle, T., Dohlman, H. G., Bolanowski, M. A., Sigal, I. S., Yang-Fing, T. L., Francke, V., Caron, M. G. and Lefkowitz, R. J. (1987). cDNA for the human β_2-adrenergic receptor: a protein with multiple membrane spanning domains and encoded by a gene whose chromosomal location is shared with that of the receptor for platelet-derived growth factor. *Proc. Natl. Acad. Sci. USA*, **84**, 46–50
9. Tota, M. R., Candelore, M. R., Dixon, R. A. F. and Strader, C. D. (1991). Biophysical and genetic analysis of the ligand binding site of the β-adrenoceptor. *Trends Pharmacol. Sci.*, **12**, 4–6
10. Gilman, A. G. (1987). G-proteins: transducers of receptor-generated signals. *Ann. Rev. Biochem.*, **56**, 615–49

11. Herbette, L. G., Trumbore, M., Chester, D. W. and Katz, A. M. (1988). Possible molecular basis for the pharmacokinetics and pharmacodynamics of three membrane-active drugs: propranolol, nimodipine and amiodarone. *J. Mol. Cell. Cardiol.*, **20**, 373–8
12. Brittain, R. T. (1990). Approaches to a long-acting, selective β_2-adrenoceptor stimulant. *Lung*, **168**, 111–14
13. Brittain, R. T., Jack, D. and Sumner, M. J. (1988). Further studies on the long duration of action of salmeterol, a new selective β_2-stimulant bronchodilator. *J. Pharm. Pharmacol.*, **40**, 93P
14. Coleman, R. A., Johnson, M., Nials, A. T. and Sumner, M. J. (1990). Salmeterol, but not formoterol, persists at β_2-adrenoceptors *in vitro. Br. J. Pharmacol.*, **99**, 121P
15. Jack, D. (1991). A way of looking at agonism and antagonism: lessons from salbutamol, salmeterol and other β-adrenoceptor agonists. *Br. J. Clin. Pharmacol.*, **31**, 501–14
16. Brittain, R. T. (1989). Approaches to a long selective β_2-adrenoceptor stimulant. *Eur. Resp. J.*, **2**, 200
17. Ullman, A. and Svedmyr, N. (1990). Inhaled salmeterol improves asthma symptoms without tachyphylaxis in a two week comparison with salbutamol. *Am. Rev. Respir. Dis.*, **141**, A206
18. Johnson, M. (1991). Salmeterol: a novel drug for the treatment of asthma. *Agents and Actions*, **34**, 79–95
19. Nials, A. T., Butchers, P. R., Coleman, R. A., Johnson, M. and Vardey, C. J. (1990). Salmeterol and formoterol, are they both long-acting β_2-adrenoceptor agonists? *Br. J. Pharmacol.*, **99**, 120P
20. Buckner, C. K. and Abel, P. (1974). Studies on the effects of the enantiomers of soterenol, trimetoquinol and salbutamol on β-adrenergic receptors of isolated guinea-pig atria and trachea. *J. Pharm. Exp. Ther.*, **189**, 616–25
21. Brittain, R. T., Farmer, J. B. and Marshall, R. J. (1973). Some observations on the β-adrenoceptor agonist properties of the isomers of salbutamol. *Br. J. Pharamcol.*, **48**, 144–7
22. Barker, R. C., Coleman, R. A., Dahl, M. R., Nials, A. T. and Vardey, C. J. (1992). Do salmeterol and formoterol possess agonist activity at atypical β-adrenoceptors in guinea-pig gastric fundus? *Br. J. Pharmacol.*, **106**, 87P
23. Ball, D. I., Brittain, R. T., Coleman, R. A., Denyer, L. H., Jack, D., Johnson, M., Lunts, L. H. C., Nials, A. T., Sheldrick, K. E. and Skidmore, I. F. (1991).

Salmeterol: a novel, long-acting β_2-adrenoceptor agonist: characterisation of pharmacological activity *in vitro* and *in vivo*. *Br. J. Pharmacol.*, **104**, 665–71

24. Johnson, M. (1991). The preclinical pharmacology of salmeterol: bronchodilator effects. *Eur. Respir. Rev.*, **1**, 253–6
25. Ball, D. I., Coleman, R. A., Denyer, L. H., Nials, A. T. and Sheldrick, K. E. (1987). Bronchodilator activity of salmeterol, a long-acting β_2-adrenoceptor agonist. *Br. J. Pharmacol.*, **92**, 746P
26. Ullman, A. and Svedmyr, N. (1988). Salmeterol, a new long-acting inhaled β_2-adrenoceptor agonist: comparison with salbutamol in adult asthmatic patients. *Thorax*, **43**, 674–8
27. Sandström, T. and Wallin, A. (1991). Rapid onset and long duration of bronchodilation with inhaled formoterol dry powder. *Am. Rev. Respir. Dis.*, **143**, A647
28. Butchers, P. R., Skidmore, I. F., Vardey, C. J. and Wheeldon, A. (1980). Characterisation of the receptor mediating the anti-asthmatic effects of β-adrenoceptor agonist in human lung tissue *in vitro*. *Br. J. Pharmacol.*, **71**, 663–7
29. Butchers, P. R., Fullarton, I. R., Skidmore, I. F., Thompson, L. E., Vardey, C. J. and Wheeldon, A. (1979). A comparison of the anti-anaphylactic activities of salbutamol and disodium cromoglycate in the rat mast cell and in human lung tissue. *Br. J. Pharmacol.*, **67**, 23–32
30. Butchers, P. R., Vardey, C. J. and Johnson, M. (1991). Salmeterol: a potent and long-acting inhibitor of inflammatory mediator release from human lung. *Br. J. Pharmacol.*, **104**, 672–6
31. Howarth, P. H., Dunham, S. R., Lee, T., Kay, A. B., Church, M. K. and Holgate, S. T. (1985). Influence of albuterol, cromolyn sodium and ipratropium bromide on the airway and circulating mediator responses to allergen bronchial provoction in asthma. *Am. Rev. Respir. Dis.*, **132**, 986–92
32. Minnear, F. L., DeMichele, M. A., Moon, D. G., Rieder, C. L. and Fenton, J. W. (1989). Isoproterenol reduces thrombin-induced pulmonary endothelial permeability *in vitro*. *Am. J. Physiol.*, **257**, H1613–23
33. Tokuyama, K., Lotvall, J. O., Löfdahl, C. G., Barnes, P. J. and Chung, K. F. (1991). Inhaled formoterol inhibits histamine-induced airflow obstruction and airway microvascular leakage. *Eur. J. Pharmacol.*, **193**, 35–9
34. Whelan, C. J. and Johnson, M. (1990). The anti-inflammatory effects of inhaled salmeterol and salbutamol in guinea-pig lung. *Br. J. Pharmacol.*, **101**, 528P
35. Whelan, C. J. and Johnson, M. (1991). Salmeterol, but not salbutamol, has anti-inflammatory activity in guinea-pig skin. *Br. J. Pharmacol.*, **102**, 95P

36. Rusznak, C., Sapsford, R. J., Devalia, J. L. and Davies, R. J. (1991). The influence of salbutamol and salmeterol on ciliary beat frequency of cultured human bronchial epithelial cells. *Thorax*, **46**, 782P
37. Johnson, M. (1990). The pharmacology of salmeterol *Lung*, **168**, 115–19
38. Baker, A. J. and Fuller, R. W. (1990). Anti-inflammatory effects of salmeterol on human alveolar macrophages. *Am. Rev. Respir. Dis.*, **141**, A394
39. Whelan, C. J. and Johnson, M. (1992). Inhibition by salmeterol of increased vascular permeability and granulocyte accumulation in guinea-pig lung and skin. *Br. J. Pharmacol.*, **105**, 831–8
40. Anderson, G. P. (1991). Pharmacology of formoterol: an innovative bronchodilator. *Agents and Actions*, **34**, 97–115
41. Nials, A. T., Whelan, C. J. and Vardey, C. J. (1991). Salmeterol inhibits neutrophil accumulation in rat lung. *Br. J. Pharmacol.*, **104**, 294P
42. Twentyman, O. P., Finnerty, I. P., Harris, A., Palmer, J. and Holgate, S. T. (1990). Protection against allergen-induced asthma by salmeterol. *Lancet*, **336**, 1338–42
43. Diaz, P., Gonzalez, M. C., Galleguillas, F. R., Ancic, P., Cromwell, O., Shepherd, D., Durham, S. R., Gleich, G. J. and Kay, A. B. (1989). Leukocytes and mediators in bronchoalveolar lavage during allergen-induced late-phase asthmatic reactions. *Am. Rev. Respir. Dis.*, **139**, 1383–9
44. Cockcroft, D. W. and Murdock, K. Y. (1987). Comparative effects of inhaled salbutamol sodium cromoglycate and beclomethasone dipropionate on allergen-induced early asthmatic responses, late asthmatic and increased bronchial hyper-reactivity to histamine. *J. Allergol. Clin. Immunol.*, **79**, 734–40
45. Fuller, R. W. (1991). Anti-inflammatory effects of salmeterol. In *Salmeterol: A Reappraisal of Asthma Management*, pp. 18–19. (Oxford: Medicines Group)
46. Palmqvist, M., Löwhagen, O., Balder, B., Melander, B., Svedmyr, N. and Wåhlander, L. (1989). Prevention of late asthmatic reaction by salbutamol and formoterol. *Eur. Resp. J.*, **8**, 768
47. Grönneberg, R. and Zetterström, O. (1990). Inhibition of anti-IgE induced skin responses in normals by formoterol, a new β_2-adrenoceptor agonist, and terbutaline: effect on the late phase reaction. *Allergy*, **45**, 340–6
48. Dahl, R., Pedersen, B. and Venge, P. (1991). Bronchoalveolar lavage studies. *Eur. Respir. Rev.*, **1**, 272–75
49. Howarth, P. H. (1991). The investigation of the non-bronchodilator properties of asthma therapics *in vivo*. *Eur. Respir. J.*, **4**, 399S

DISCUSSION

Prof. J. Barnes (London) I think one of the very important issues that now needs to be addressed is tachyphylaxis and down-regulation of non-airway smooth muscle effects of β-agonists. Much of the debate about β-agonists now is not whether or not they are bronchodilators but what other actions they have. From the studies we have done on other systems outside airway smooth muscle, I think we would conclude that tachyphylaxis develops extremely rapidly.

Have you looked at tachyphylaxis of some of these other effects you discussed, such as the microvascular leakage effect and effects on ciliary beat frequency, for example?

Dr M. Johnson We have looked at tachyphylaxis in some but not all of these systems. In the guinea-pig lung model looking at vascular permeability, there is no evidence of tachyphylaxis to the inhibitory effects of salmeterol. In terms of inflammatory cell accumulation effects, both in the skin and in the lung again there is no evidence following up to 5 days' dosing with salmeterol.

I cannot speak for Dr Davies' experiments with bronchial epithelium, but I believe they are with the β-agonist present in the culture medium for 24 h.

Dr D. Raeburn (Rhône–Poulenc Rorer, Dagenham) Your data show quite clearly that salmeterol inhibits eosinophil accumulation into the lung. You will be aware of the study by Sanjar who showed that there was no correlation between the number of eosinophils and the state of activation or hyper-reactivity in his model and yours. Are there any data relating to the effect of salmeterol on the activation state of the eosinophil rather than on eosinophil number?

Dr M. Johnson I think this is a very important question. These studies are being carried out at the moment. All I can say now is that in the antigen challenge model there is a circulating eosinophilia. We see no effect of salmeterol on circulating eosinophil numbers, which remain elevated, but there is an effect on the number of cells that infiltrate through to the airway lumen. We are now looking at the activation state of these cells in terms of histology and the mediators they are releasing. This should provide the answer to the question.

Prof. Sir James Black (UK) With regard to the function of mast cells, is it your view that although they are widely distributed mast cells play no physiological role? Is it your judgement that prolonged activation of β-receptors would have no downside on physiological function?

Dr M. Johnson It is important to differentiate in this context the lung mast cell from extrapulmonary mast cells. At one stage, the lung mast cell *was* believed to be the key in asthma. This was clearly naive then as it is now, and the failure of so-called 'mast-cell stabilizing drugs' led to a swing of opinion away from the mast cell as an important cell. I think we are now beginning to see that the mast cell may indeed play a role in the disease – but it is clearly not the only cell involved. It requires studies similar to those carried out by Prof. Holgate's group with salbutamol to demonstrate *in vivo* in the asthmatic patient that mast cell-specific mediators can be influenced by anti-asthma drugs such as β-agonists, when they are delivered at therapeutic doses by the inhaled route. By that type of approach, I believe it will be possible to evaluate how important the mast cell really is.

Is there any downside to inhibiting mast cells? All I can say is that in salmeterol we have a potent, long-lasting, inhibitor of mast cell function. No adverse effects have been observed in all the toxicological studies that have been carried out with very high doses that would lead to the suggestion that inhibition of mast cells is a problem.

3

β_2-Agonists and the mast cell

C. P. Page

The involvement of the mast cell in the pathogenesis of allergic asthma has been promulgated since the discovery in the 1960s that sodium cromoglycate was clinically useful in the treatment of asthma[1] and that this drug had the pharmacological property of being able to inhibit the release of mediators from chopped human lung and rat peritoneal mast cells[2] induced by antigen–antibody interactions. Such observations led to the concept that this drug worked in asthma via its ability to act as a mast cell stabilizer, which has subsequently become dogma. This hypothesis, however, led to the development by the pharmaceutical industry of a wide range of novel chemical entities having the ability to stabilize mast cells, all of considerably greater potency than sodium cromoglycate, and, whilst many of these agents were developed as far as clinical trials and were clearly demonstrated to be capable of inhibiting acute allergic bronchoconstriction, which is undoubtedly secondary to the release of mast-cell-derived spasmogens prostaglandin D_2, histamine and leukotriene C_4 (reviewed in reference 3), none of them proved to be of benefit in the treatment of asthma (reviewed in references 4–6), raising doubts about the central role of the mast cell in asthma[7].

In early studies investigating the pharmacological manipulation of mast cell degranulation, it became apparent that whilst sodium cromoglycate was often used as the 'gold standard' mast cell stabilizing agent, its ability to inhibit mediator release from chopped human lung was trivial in comparison with drugs capable of stimulating adenylate cyclase, such as the β-agonists[8]. Furthermore, the non-selective β-agonist isoprenaline has been recognized since the 1960s to be capable of inhibiting histamine release from leukocytes[9]. More recent studies with highly purified human lung mast cell populations have adequately confirmed these original findings and extended them to show that this inhibitory effect on mediator release is via activation of β_2-receptors on the human lung mast cell and that in comparison to the

β_2-selective agonists, salbutamol[10,11], or salmeterol[12], sodium cromoglycate is almost inactive at inhibiting the release of histamine from purified human lung mast cells[8,10,11]. Moreover, clinically useful doses of β_2-agonists have been shown to inhibit the release of histamine into the circulation of asthmatics undergoing allergen provocation suggesting that this pharmacological property of β_2-agonists may well contribute to the recognized ability of these drugs to inhibit allergen-induced bronchoconstriction in addition to the obvious bronchodilator properties of such drugs[13]. Whilst recent clinical studies have also reported that the failure of salmeterol to inhibit the allergen-induced rise in urinary leukotriene E_4 argues against this pharmacological property of β_2-agonists occurring *in vivo*, these authors have not actually demonstrated that the increased leukotriene E_4 actively derives from lung mast cells[14].

Despite the proliferation of literature on mast cell biology over the last two decades, heparin and related proteoglycans are mast cell products that have not received a great deal of attention. These highly anionic molecules have only been ascribed the function of binding histamine within mast cell granules, but, there is now accumulating evidence that these molecules may act as natural anti-inflammatory molecules and thus have a far greater role in the pathogenesis of allergic diseases than was previously thought. Studies dating back to the 1920s have reported that heparin can inhibit the features of anaphylaxis[15] and clinical reports have also appeared in the literature showing that heparin is capable of modulating allergic responses in man, both in the skin, and the respiratory system[16–18]. It is also of interest that an increase in the circulating levels of an endogenous 'heparin-like material' has been shown to be present in the plasma of allergic subjects[19]. Furthermore, a radiographic analysis of 50 adult asthmatics has revealed that such subjects have less calcification of major arterial blood vessels when compared with age- and sex-matched control subjects, and these differences have been attributed to higher levels of circulating 'heparin-like material'[20].

Over recent years, a case has been made for the eosinophil as an important cell in initiating the tissue damage characterizing various allergic diseases (e.g. the epithelial desquamation observed in the lungs of asthmatics)[21]. This tissue damage has been suggested to be mediated in part via the release of cytotoxic mediators such as major basic protein, eosinophil cationic protein and eosinophil peroxidase[21,22]. These cationic proteins are known to be neutralized by the anionic heparin, and heparin affinity columns have been used to purify many of these cationic proteins. Furthermore, heparin has been demonstrated to inhibit the epithelial damage induced by some of these cationic proteins[22]. Interestingly, it has recently been reported that another cationic protein, platelet factor 4 is a chemotactic agent for human eosinophils[23], and it has long been recognized for its ability to bind heparin[24]. It is therefore plausible that endogenous heparin could be released to limit the extent of eosinophil recruitment into sites of allergic inflammation and to limit the extent of tissue damage induced by leukocyte-derived cationic proteins. Certainly heparin has been shown to inhibit the ability of antigen–antibody reactions and the ether-linked phospholipid, platelet activating factor to induce eosinophil infiltration into the lung tissue of experimental animals[25]. This could be due to a direct effect of heparin on the eosinophil as has been described with neutrophils[26] or be secondary to an effect on the adhesion and diapedesis of these cells from blood vessels by increasing the negative charge on the endothelial cell lining[27]. Likewise, heparin has also been shown to inhibit the increased vascular permeability induced by a wide range of agonists acting via specific receptors located on the vascular endothelial cells, possibly via a non-specific increase in the negative charge on the endothelial cells[28].

There is now a growing interest in the involvement of lymphocytes in the pathogenesis of allergic asthma[29]. It is therefore of interest that recent studies have suggested that heparin can inhibit lymphocyte activation[30,31] and trafficking[32] and is capable of inhibiting delayed hypersensitivity responses[33,34], recognized as being a lymphocyte-driven inflammatory response. The mechanism whereby heparin is able to inhibit these responses is unclear but it has been reported that a similar anti-inflammatory effect can be obtained by using heparin-like molecules devoid of anticoagulant activity[34], suggesting that this effect is not simply due to inhibition of the coagulation cascade.

Mast cells have also been described as having other properties that could be interpreted as being anti-inflammatory. For instance, following the intradermal administration of human eosinophil-derived major basic protein into human skin, this material is rapidly incorporated into mast cells, possibly to neutralize its charge and therefore limit its toxic activity[35]. Furthermore, mast cell proteases have been shown to have a regulatory role in degrading sensory neuropeptides[36], implicated in a number of inflammatory conditions and, more recently, the histamine released from mast cells has been shown to switch off cytokine production in mast cells via the activation of histamine type 2 receptors[37].

Asthma can certainly now be considered a chronic inflammatory disease and following each exposure to allergen that results in tissue damage, it is likely that the body will try to repair such damaged tissue. This is most probably evident in the asthmatic lung as the thickened basement membrane which is now thought to be related to subepithelial fibrosis[38], the presence of myofibroblasts[39] and collagen deposition[40]. Additionally it has been recognized that asthma is characterized by a thickened smooth muscle layer[41]. Recent studies using histological analysis of material biopsied from the lungs of asthmatics have revealed that these changes appear very early in the disease and are not just features of patients with chronic asthma[38]. Furthermore, even following chronic treatment with inhaled glucocorticoids, the thickness of the basement membrane is not reduced, even though such therapy reduces the number of inflammatory cells present in the biopsies and the extent of epithelial damage[42]. It is also noteworthy that 10 years of treatment with glucocorticoids does not reduce airway hyper-responsiveness completely, despite reducing the number of inflammatory cells present in the airways[43]. Since others have suggested that airway wall thickening may account for bronchial hyper-responsiveness on geometric grounds[44], such clinical observations may reflect that once these anatomical changes have appeared they may not be reversible, even with the most aggressive therapy currently available. One of the interests in the biology of proteoglycans is because of their ability to inhibit both fibroblast proliferation[45] and smooth muscle thickening, although the latter has only been demonstrated with vascular[46] and intestinal smooth muscle[47]. Additionally, heparin has been demonstrated to inhibit the vascular remodelling normally seen *in vivo* following chronic hypoxia[48]. It would therefore seem prudent to investigate the role of proteoglycans in the control of airway smooth muscle thickening and myofibroblast proliferation in the lung.

It is my hypothesis that allergic subjects degranulate mast cells in response to allergen exposure to release histamine and other spasmogens to induce bronchoconstriction as a primitive defence mechanism to limit antigen burden[7]. Recent evidence has supported this hypothesis as experimental inhibition of the acute bronchoconstriction induced by antigen challenge of allergic animals by pretreatment with a β_2-agonist results in a far greater influx of inflammatory cells into the lung 24 h later than if the animals are allowed to undergo bronchoconstriction[49,50]. A clinical corollary exists in that allergic asthmatic patients undergoing acute bronchoconstriction only following allergen challenge have a far greater release of mast cell-derived spasmogens into bronchoalveolar lavage fluid 5 min after challenge than patients who subsequently go on to have a late asthmatic response[51]. Furthermore, pretreatment of allergic asthmatics who normally only undergo acute bronchospasm following allergen challenge, with a histamine type 1 antagonist[52] or the β_2-agonist rimiterol hydrobromide[53] results in such patients subsequently undergoing a late asthmatic response following allergen challenge. These observations may be seen as mast cell degranulation occurring to limit allergen burden and that by inhibiting this process, the disease process is actually modified in an adverse way. Heparin has also been shown to inhibit allergen-induced bronchospasm[54] and the release of heparin by mast cells may also have been developed teliologically to serve to limit the acute inflammatory response initiated to deal with the inhaled antigen by inhibiting eosinophil infiltration and neutralizing the toxic effects of released cationic proteins[7]. Released heparin may also serve to limit the extent of the subsequent repair process by controlling the deposition of smooth muscle or fibroblasts[7]. In this way the degranulation of mast cells can be considered teliologically as a beneficial event designed to limit antigen burden and provide a homeostatic mechanism to limit self tissue damage. The ability of β_2-agonists to inhibit allergen-induced release of proteoglycans from human lung mast cells[55] could therefore potentially lead to an inhibition of this endogenous homeostatic mechanism, and thus the regular use of β_2-agonists may actually allow both a chronic increase in allergen burden, and thus an increase in airways inflammation which subsequently results in the appearance of excess deposition of scar tissue. The chronic appearance of 'scar' tissue may in turn be responsible for the persistent airways hyper-responsiveness that appears to be resistant to even glucocorticoid therapy[42,43]. The regular use of this class of drugs may therefore be accelerating the disease process in a manner analogous to that suggested to occur with the regular use of non-steroidal anti-inflammatory drugs in patients with arthritis[56]. It is also worth considering that by the regular use of early sympathomimetic therapy we may therefore be actually allowing a self-limiting disease to become a chronic disease having an irreversible component.

Whilst this hypothesis remains to be fully proven, the clinical studies showing that regular treatment with β_2-agonists actually exacerbates one of the underlying features of the disease, namely bronchial hyper-responsiveness[57–62], the recent suggestion that regular use of β_2-agonists may actually be a risk factor for death[63,64], and the very real possibility that the regular use of β_2-agonists may actually allow an increased antigen burden to patients[7,49,50,53] should not be ignored and merit considerable further attention. If it is true that the anatomical changes resulting from excess repair cannot be reversed even by chronic treatment with inhaled glucocorticoids, then the emphasis for future asthma research should be in the area of identifying subjects as early as possible in life who are at risk from developing allergic diseases and initiating the earlier treatment of these subjects with prophylactic antiasthma drugs rather than with early symptomatic therapy as now being suggested by most Clinical Societies in their Guidelines to Management.

It remains important that clinicians and scientists alike err on the side of caution when considering the recent suggestions that novel long-acting β_2-agonists such as salmeterol may actually be anti-inflammatory as well as bronchodilators by virtue of their ability to inhibit mast cell degranulation[65]. The suggestion that β_2-agonists are anti-inflammatory via this mechanism in addition to causing obvious bronchodilatation is still unproven and in fact contrary evidence exists[49,50]. More prospective trials are required to evaluate the long-term effects of β_2-agonists on the outcome of asthma, and such clinical studies have clearly revealed that regular use of β_2-agonists actually gives worse overall control than when β_2-agonists are used *pro re nata*[59,66], or than regular treatment with glucocorticoids[67]. The regular use of β_2-agonists may have recently been awarded the all clear with regard to risk of death by the Committee of Safety of Medicines but the contribution of this class of drug to the worrying and continuing increase in morbidity associated with this disease still requires further investigation.

REFERENCES

1. Cox, J. S. C. (1971). Disodium cromoglycate, mode of actions and possible relevance to the clinical use of the drug. *Br. J. Dis. Chest*, **65**, 189–204
2. Cox, J. S. C. (1967). Disodium cromoglycate (FPL 670) (Intal): a specific inhibitor of reaginic antibody/antigen mechanisms. *Nature (London)*, **216**, 1328
3. Minshall, E. M. and Page, C. P. (1992). Mast cells and the lung. In Foreman, J. (ed.) *Immunopharmacology of Mast Cells and Basophils*, in press. (London: Academic Press)
4. Auty, R. M. (1986). The clinical development of a new agent for the treatment of airways inflammation, nedocromil sodium (Tilade). *Eur. J. Respir. Dis.*, **69**, Suppl. 147, 120–31

5. Garland, L. G. (1991). Pharmacology of prophylactic antiasthma drugs. In Barnes, P. J. and Page, C. P. (eds.) *Pharmacology of Asthma*, pp. 261–90. (Heidelberg: Springer-Verlag)
6. Stokes, T. C. and Morley, J. (1981). Prospects for an oral intal. *Br. J. Dis. Chest*, **75**, 1–14
7. Page, C. P. (1991). One explanation of the asthma paradox: inhibition of natural anti-inflammatory mechanism by β_2-agonists. *Lancet*, **337**, 717–20
8. Butchers, P. R., Fullerton, J. R., Skidmore, I. F., Thompson, L. E., Vardey, C. E. and Wheldon, A. (1979). A comparison of the anti-anaphylactic actions of salbutamol and disodium cromoglycate in the rat, the rat mast cell and human lung tissue. *Br. J. Pharmacol.*, **67**, 23–32
9. Lichtenstein, L. M. and Margolis, S. (1968). Histamine release *in vitro*: inhibition by catecholamines and methylxanthines. *Science*, **161**, 902–3
10. Church, M. K. and Hiroi, J. (1987). Inhibition of IgE dependent histamine release from human dispersed mast cells by antiallergic drugs and salbutamol. *Br. J. Pharmacol.*, **90**, 421–9
11. Church, M. K. and Young, K. D. (1983). The characteristics of inhibition of histamine release from human lung fragments by sodium cromoglycate, salbutamol and chlorpromazine. *Br. J. Pharmacol.*, **78**, 671–9
12. Butchers, P. R., Vardey, C. J. and Johnson, M. (1991). Salmeterol: a potent and long-acting inhibitor of inflammatory mediator release from human lung. *Br. J. Pharmacol.*, **104**, 672–6
13. Howarth, P. H., Durham, S. R., Lee, T. H., Kay, A. B., Church, M. K. and Holgate, S. T. (1985). Influence of albuterol, cromolyn sodium and ipatropium bromide on the airway and circulatory mediator responses to allergen bronchial provocation in asthma. *Am. Rev. Respir. Dis.*, **132**, 986–92
14. Taylor, I. K., O'Shaughnessey, K. M., Choudry, N. B., Adachi, M., Palmer, J. B. D. and Fuller, R. W. (1992). A comparative study in atopic subjects with asthma of the effects of salmeterol and salbutamol on allergen induced bronchoconstriction, increase in airway reactivity and increase in urinary leukotriene E4 excretion. *J. Allergy Clin. Immunol.*, **89**, 578–83
15. Van der Carr, F. R. and Williams, O. B. (1928). Further studies on the influence of heparin on anaphylactic shock in the guinea pig. *J. Immunol.*, **15**, 13–20
16. Bowler, S. (1988). Heparin, allergy, mast cells and asthma. In Conference documentation, *Heparin and Related Polysaccharides – New Directions for Old Drugs*. (London, December 29/30: IBC Technical Services)
17. Dahl, Sv. (1962). Heparin und asthma. *Tuberkulose*, **118**, 255–62

18. Dolowitz, D. A. and Dougherty, T. F. (1965). The use of heparin in the control of allergies. *Ann. Allergy*, **23**, 309–13
19. Lasser, E. C., Simon, R. A., Lyon, S. G., Hamblin, A. W. and Stein, R. (1987). Heparin-like anticoagulants in asthma. *Allergy*, **42**, 619–25
20. Lasser, E. C., Berry, C. and Kortmann, K. (1987). Diminished atherosclerotic arterial calcifications in asthma. A possible role for elevated endogenous heparin like material. *Allergy*, **42**, 549–52
21. Dahl, R., Venge, P. and Fredens, K. (1988). Eosinophils. In Barnes, P. J., Rodger, I. W. and Thomson, N. C. (eds.) *Asthma Basic Mechanisms and Clinical Management*, pp. 115–29. (London: Academic Press)
22. Motojima, S., Frigas, E., Lowgering, D. A. and Gleich, G. J. (1989). Toxicity of eosinophil cationic proteins for guinea pig tracheal epithelium *in vitro*. *Am. Rev. Respir. Dis.*, **139**, 801–5
23. Chihara, J., Fukuda, K., Yasuba, H., Kishigari, N., Sugihara, R., Kubo, H. and Nakajima, S. (1988). Platelet factor 4 enhances eosinophil IgG and IgEFc receptors and has eosinophil chemotactic activity. *Am. Rev. Respir. Dis.*, **137**, A421
24. Block, P. E., Luscomb, M., Marshall, S. E., Pepper, D. S. and Holbrook, J. J. (1980). The multiple complexes formed by the interaction of platelet factor 4 with heparin. *Biochem. J.*, **191**, 769–76
25. Seeds, E. A. M. and Page, C. P. (1992). The effect of heparin and related molecules of PAF and antigen-induced eosinophil infiltration in guinea pigs. *Am. Rev. Respir. Dis.*, **145**, A697
26. Matzner, Y., Marx, G., Drexler, R. and Eldor, E. (1984). The inhibitory effect of heparin and related glycoaminoglycans on neutrophil chemotaxis. *Thromb. Haemostas.*, **52**, 134–7
27. Doutrempuich, C., Touslemonde, F., De Seze, O., Pereira, F., Anne, M. C. and Doutrempuich, F. (1987). Influence of heparin and a low molecular weight heparin fraction on the leukocytes in an experimental venous thrombosis model. *J. Leukocyte Biol.*, **42**, 628–31
28. Carr, J. (1979). The anti-inflammatory action of heparins: heparin as an antagonist to histamine, bradykinin and prostaglandin E. *Thromb. Res.*, **16**, 507–16
29. Robinson, D. S., Hamid, Q., Ying, S., Tsicopoulos, A., Barkans, J., Berthy, A. M., Corrigan, C., Durham, S. R. and Kay, A. B. (1992). Predominant TH2-like bronchoalveolar T lymphocyte population in atopic asthma. *N. Engl. J. Med.*, **326**, 298–304

30. Frieri, M. and Metcalf, D. D. (1983). Analysis of the effect of mast cell granules on lymphocyte blastogenesis in the absence and presence of mitogens. Identification of heparin as a granule associated suppressor factor. *J. Immunol.*, **131**, 1942–7
31. Gorski, A., Wasik, M., Nowaczyk, M. and Korczak-Kowalska, G. (1991). Immunological aspects of heparin. *FASEB J.*, **5**, 2287–91
32. Willenborg, D. O. and Parish, C. R. (1988). Inhibition of allergic encephalomyelitis in rats by treatment with sulphated polysaccharides. *J. Immunol.*, **140**, 3401–5
33. Cohen, S., Benacerraf, B., McCluskey, R. T. and Ovary, Z. (1967). Effect of anticoagulants on delayed hypersensitivity. *J. Immunol.*, **98**, 351–7
34. Sy, M. S., Scneeburger, E., Greene, M. I. *et al.* (1983). Inhibition of delayed type hypersensitivity by heparin depleted of anticoagulant activity. *Cell. Immunol.*, **82**, 23–32
35. Butterfield, J. H., Weiler, D., Peterson, E. A., Gleich, G. J. and Leiferman, K. M. (1990). Sequestration of eosinophil major basic protein in human mast cells. *Lab. Invest.*, **62**, 77–86
36. Caughey, G. H. (1989). Roles of mast cell tryptase and chymase in airway function. *Am. J. Physiol.*, **257**, L39–46
37. Vannier, E., Miller, L. C. and Dinarello, C. A. (1991). Histamine suppresses gene expression and synthesis of TNFα via histamine H2 receptors. *J. Exp. Med.*, **174**, 281–4
38. Roche, W. R., Beasley, R., Williams, J. H. and Holgate, S. T. (1989). Subepithelial fibrosis in the bronchi of asthmatics. *Lancet*, **1**, 520–4
39. Brewster, C. E. P., Howarth, P. H., Djukanovic, R. *et al.* (1990). Myofibroblasts and sub-epithelial fibrosis in bronchial asthma. *Am. J. Respir. Cell Mol. Biol.*, **3**, 507–11
40. Beasley, R., Roche, W. R., Roberts, A. and Holgate, S. T. (1989). Cellular events in the bronchi of asthmatics. *Am. Rev. Respir. Dis.*, **139**, 806–17
41. Ebina, M., Yaegashi, H., Chiba, R., Takahashi, T., Motomiya, M. and Tanemura, M. (1990). Hyperreactive site in the airway tree of asthmatic patients revealed by thickening of bronchial muscles: a morphometric study. *Am. Rev. Respir. Dis.*, **141**, 1327–32
42. Jeffrey, P. K., Godfrey, R. W., Adelroth, E. and Johansson, S. A. (1990). Effects of treatment on airway mucosal cell infiltrate and thickening of reticular basement membrane in asthma. *Am. Rev. Respir. Dis.*, **141**, A500

43. Lungren, R., Soderberg, M., Horstedt, P. and Stenling, R. (1988). Morphological studies on bronchial mucosal biopsies from asthmatics before and after 10 years of treatment with inhaled steroids. *Eur. Respir. J.*, **1**, 883–9

44. James, A. L., Pare, P. D. and Hogg, J. C. (1989). The mechanisms of airway narrowing in asthma. *Am. Rev. Respir. Dis.*, **139**, 242–6

45. San Antonio, J. D., Lander, R. D., Wright, T. C. and Karnovsky, M. J. (1992). Heparin inhibits the attachment and growth of Balb/c-3T3 fibroblasts on collagen substrata. *J. Cell Physiol.*, **150**, 8–16

46. Benitz, W. E., Kelly, R. T., Anderson, C. M., Lorant, D. E. and Bernfield, M. (1990). Endothelial heparin sulphate proteoglycan 1. Inhibitory effects on smooth muscle proliferation. *Am. J. Respir. Cell Mol. Biol.*, **2**, 13–24

47. Graham, M. F., Drucker, D. E., Perr, H. A., Diegelmann, R. F. and Ehrlich, H. P. (1987). Heparin modulated human intestinal smooth muscle proliferation protein synthesis and lattice contraction. *Gastroenterology*, **93**, 801–9

48. Hales, C. A., Kradin, R. L., Brardsetter, R. D. and Zhu, Y. S. (1983). Impairment of hypoxic pulmonary artery remodelling by heparin in mice. *Am. Rev. Respir. Dis.*, **128**, 747–51

49. Manzini, S., Pettetti, F., Abelli, L., Evangelista, S., Giachetti, A., Seeds, E. A. M. and Page, C. P. (1992). Isbufylline a new xanthine derivative inhibits airway hyperresponsiveness and inflammation in guinea pigs. *Br. J. Pharmacol.*, in press

50. Sanjar, S., Aoki, S., Kristersson, A., Smith, D. and Morley, J. (1990). Antigen challenge induces pulmonary airway eosinophil accumulation and airway hyperreactivity in sensitised guinea pigs. *Br. J. Pharmacol.*, **99**, 679–86

51. Wenzel, S E., Westcott, J. Y. and Larsen, G. L. (1991). Bronchoalveolar lavage fluid mediator levels 5 minutes after allergen challenge in atopic subjects with asthma: relationship to the development of late asthmatic responses. *J. Allergy Clin. Immunol.*, **87**, 540–8

52. Lai, C. K. W., Beasley, R. and Holgate, S. T. (1989). The effect of an increase in inhaled allergen dose after terfenadine on the occurrence and magnitude of the late asthmatic response. *Clin. Exp. Allergy*, **19**, 209–16

53. Lai, C. K. W., Twentyman, O. P. and Holgate, S. T. (1987). The effect of an increase in inhaled allergen dose after inhaled rimeterol hydrobromide and the occurrence and magnitude of the late asthmatic response and the associated changes in non-specific bronchial responsiveness. *Am. Rev. Respir. Dis.*, **140**, 917–23

54. Ahmed, T., Abraham, W. M. and D'Brot, J. (1992). Effects of inhaled heparin on immunologic and nonimmunologic bronchoconstrictor responses in sheep. *Am. Rev. Respir. Dis.*, **145**, 566–70

55. Green, W. F., Konnaris, K. and Woolcock, A. J. (1992). The effect of salbutamol., feneterol and sodium cromoglycate on the release of heparin from sensitized human lung fragments challenged with *D. pteronyssinus* allergen. *Aust. N. Z. J. Med.*, in press

56. Rashad, S., Revell, P., Hemmingway, A., Low, F., Rainsford, K. and Walker, F. (1989). Effect of nonsteroidal antiinflammatory drugs on the course of osteoarthritis. *Lancet*, **2**, 519–22

57. Kerrebijn, K. F., Van Essen-Zandvliet, E. E. M. and Neijens, J. H. (1987). Effect of long term treatment with inhaled corticosteroids and beta-agonists on the bronchial responsiveness in children with asthma. *J. Allergy Clin. Immunol.*, **79**, 653–9

58. Kraan, J., Koeter, G. H., van der Mark, Th. W., Sluiter, H. J. and De Vries, K. (1985). Changes in bronchial hyperreactivity induced by 4 weeks of treatment with antiasthmatic drugs in patients with allergic asthma: a comparison between budesonide and terbutaline. *J. Allergy Clin. Immunol.*, **76**, 628–36

59. Sears, M. R., Taylor, D. R., Print, G. G., Lake, D. C., Qingqing, L., Flannery, E. M., Yates, D. M., Lucas, M. K. and Herbison, G. P. (1990). Regular inhaled beta agonist treatment in bronchial asthma. *Lancet*, **336**, 1391–6

60. Vathenen, A. S., Knox, A. J., Higgins, B. G., Britton, J. R. and Tattersfield, A. E. (1988). Rebound increase in bronchial responsiveness after treatment with inhaled terbutaline. *Lancet*, **1**, 554–8

61. Van Schayck, C. P., Visch, M. B., van Herwaarden, C. L. A., Dorpeling, E. and Van Wed, C. (1990). Increased bronchial hyperresponsiveness after inhaling salbutamol during one year is not caused by desensitisation to salbutamol. *J. Allergy Clin. Immunol.*, **86**, 793–800

62. Wahedna, I., Wisniewski, A., Wong, C., Pavord, I. and Tatterfield, A. E. (1991). Airway effects of regular broxaterol and salbutamol treatment in asthmatic subjects. *Thorax*, **46**, 770P

63. Crane, S., Pearce, N., Platt, A., Burgess, C., Jackson, R., Kwong, T., Ball, M. and Beasley, R. (1989). Prescribed feneterol and death from asthma in New Zealand 1981–1983: case controlled study. *Lancet*, **1**, 917–22

64. Spitzer, W. O., Suissa, S., Ernst, P., Horwitz, R. I., Habbick, B., Cockcroft, D., Bovin, J.-F., McNutt, M., Buist, A. S. and Rebuck, A. S. (1992). Asthma death and near fatal asthma in relation to beta agonist use. *N. Engl. J. Med.*, **326**, 501–6

65. Twentyman, O. P., Finnerly, J. P., Harris, A., Palmer, J. and Holgate, S. T. (1990). Protection against allergen-induced asthma by salmeterol. *Lancet*, **336**, 1338–42
66. Van Schayck, C. P., Dorpeling, E., van Herwaarden, C. L. A., Folgerling, H., Verbeek, A. L. M., Van der Hoogen, H. J. M. and van Weel, C. (1991). Bronchodilator treatment in moderate asthma or chronic bronchitis: continuous or on demand. *Br. Med. J.*, **303**, 1428–31
67. Haahtela, T., Jarvinen, M., Kava, T., Kiviranta, K., Koskinen, S., Lehtonen, K., Nikander, K., Persson, T., Reinikainen, K., Selroos, O., Sovijarvi, A., Stenius-Aarniala, B., Svahn, T., Tammivaara, R. and Laitinen, L. A. (1991). Comparison of a β2-agonist, terbutaline, with an inhaled corticosteroid budesonide, in newly detected asthma. *N. Engl. J. Med.*, **325**, 388–92

DISCUSSION

Dr R. Fuller (Glaxo) It is an interesting hypothesis. How does the fact that Prof. Barnes has shown that the mast cell inhibition of short-acting β-agonists lasts for less than a week fit in with your hypothesis? If the effect is lost within a week of treatment, surely this means that there will not be much of a problem?

Dr C. P. Page To the best of my knowledge, no one has actually shown that *in vivo*. There are no definitive studies that show this desensitization.

Dr M. Johnson (Glaxo) In discussing the potential of heparin, it is important to recognize that for all the literature evidence that you presented there is an equal amount of evidence to show that heparin is pro-inflammatory: it increases immunoglobulin synthesis, it is a mitogen for lymphocytes, it stabilizes tryptase and increases kinin levels. The only clinical study I know that has addressed this question was carried out by Dahl in Denmark some years ago. Heparin was given to asthmatic patients, but the trial had to be terminated because they were getting worse.

Dr C. P. Page That is in contrast to two other studies of which I know. I would like to see the literature that heparin is pro-inflammatory because, as I said, with lymphocytes what matters is the dose. Low doses were used in the experiments by both Grazinsky's and the Harvard groups. I accept that *in vitro* there are higher doses of heparin which may have what you would term 'inflammatory' effects on lymphocytes, but very low doses *in vivo* –

and surprisingly even giving oral proteoglycans – will have significant immunosuppressive effects.

It is not just in this area. With the immunosuppression associated with allograft rejection and with delayed hypersensitivity, they are very low levels, equivalent to that released by the human lung.

Prof. Sir James Black (UK) I would like to congratulate Dr Page. Taking a controversial stand always takes a lot of courage. It is important to take a physiological look at problems, rather than the contemporary trend of taking the molecular route.

May I remind the audience, first, that work on mast cells really began with Reilly and Webb in the 1950s who showed that the mast cell-rich areas were all the rubbing surfaces: pleura, conjunctiva, joints, middle ear.

Secondly, these were all tissues that were damaged by practolol. Practolol was the most powerful long-lasting partial agonist that we had. If a β-agonist is given to something like mast cells, which are normally exposed to extremely low concentrations of catecholamines, they get a degree of stimulation which they never normally see. Dr Page is showing here a suggestion of what the pathological basis might be, namely, that inhibiting the mast cell removes the suppression of fibrosis. This is what happened in the eye, joints, pleura etc. (with practolol).

These are early days for salmeterol, so I beg all the clinicians looking at these patients to keep their eyes open for the practolol syndrome.

4

Adverse reactions to sympathomimetics in laboratory animals

J. Morley

INTRODUCTION

Sympathomimetics comprise the most frequently used asthma therapy. Such drugs have been selected to provide rapid symptomatic relief of airway obstruction and hence are categorized as bronchodilators. It is widely presumed that these drugs diminish airway obstruction in asthmatics by direct relaxation of airway smooth muscle, although it is now apparent that transient suppression of airway hyper-reactivity is a more plausible mechanism[1]. Neither process anticipates clinical findings that associate the use of sympathomimetics with overt airway obstruction[2], airway hyper-reactivity[3], deterioration of disease control[4], mismatch between pharmacokinetics and pharmacodynamics[5] and increased frequency of asthma death[6]; nor does relief of airway obstruction explain the improvement of clinical asthma that can arise following withdrawal of this type of therapy[7,8]. Clearly, the pharmacology of these compounds is inadequately documented.

AIRWAY HYPER-REACTIVITY

Airway hyper-reactivity is a primary determinant of acute changes in asthma symptomology, so that it is of interest to define properties of antiasthma drugs by reference to whole animal preparations in which this phenomenon is manifest. Intravenous infusion of platelet activating factor in the anaesthetized ventilated guinea-pig provides a convenient preparation[9], in which development of airway hyper-reactivity can be pre-empted by a number of established antiasthma drugs[10]. (±) Racemic-isoprenaline (rac-isoprenaline) is a noteworthy exception, since this drug augments the hyper-reactivity that develops during infusion of platelet activating factor. Exacerbation of airway hyper-reactivity was not anticipated, since acute administration of rac-isoprenaline strongly inhibits established or induced airway obstruction in this species. Hence, it became necessary to consider whether intravenous infusion of rac-isoprenaline *per se* might induce airway hyper-reactivity. Observation of the kinetics of the response to intravenous infusion of rac-isoprenaline revealed that suppression of constrictor responses to airway spasmogens is a property that, in the guinea-pig, wanes quickly to be superseded by a phase in which reactivity to airway spasmogens is heightened. Induction of airway hyper-reactivity by rac-isoprenaline is not stereospecific and this phenomenon is clearly demonstrated following intravenous infusion of either enantiomer[11]. From these observations, it may be inferred that the capacity of rac-isoprenaline to evoke increased reactivity of the airways cannot be attributed to an interaction with adrenoceptors. Further experimental analysis supports this conclusion. Thus, resolution of airway obstruction by rac-isoprenaline can be mimicked by infusion of forskolin (an adenylate cyclase activator), is suppressed by intravenous infusion of rac-propranolol, and is not affected by section of the vagus nerves; conversely, development of airway hyper-reactivity does not follow intravenous infusion of forskolin and the increased reactivity of the airways which follows intravenous infusion of rac-isoprenaline is enhanced by rac-propranolol and is pre-empted by vagal nerve section[12,13]. The net effect of intravenous infusion of rac-isoprenaline may be considered to be a summation of these two conflicting properties (Figure 1). In circumstances of endogenous constrictor tone, as in asthma, it might be expected that relief of airway obstruction due to inhalation of rac-isoprenaline could be followed by a period of obstruction, a response pattern that has been noted in patients with anomalous responses to rac-isoprenaline[2,14].

SUDDEN DEATH

Having recognized that rac-isoprenaline has an intrinsic capacity to induce airway hyper-reactivity in the guinea-pig, it is likely that expression of this property could result in death in certain circumstances. This outcome can be anticipated with some certainty, since it is well known that exposure of guinea-pigs to rac-propranolol, which produces airway hyper-reactivity by

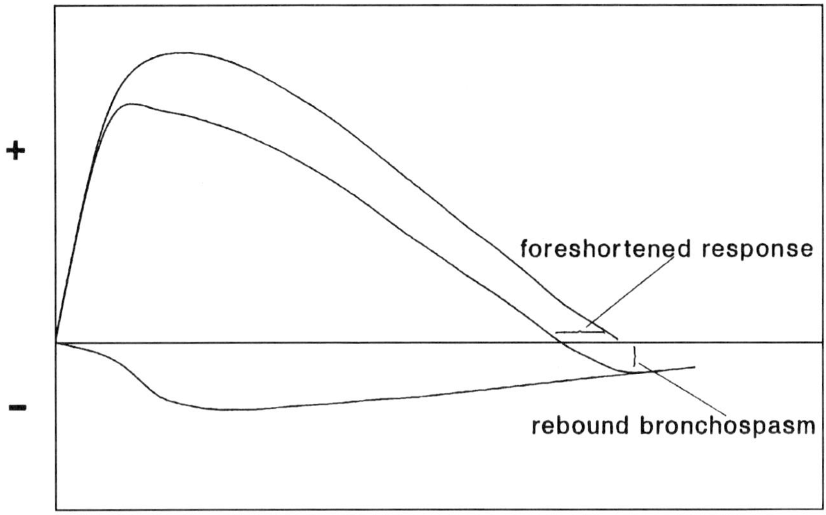

Figure 1 Diagrammatic representation of net effect of racemic β_2-selective sympathomimetics upon airway reactivity. The upper trace depicts reduction of airway responsivity to spasmogens due to activation of adrenoceptors by the L-enantiomer, whilst the lower trace depicts an increase of airway responsivity to spasmogens that results from the actions of the D-enantiomer upon vagal nerves. The net effect on airway hyper-reactivity is thereby diminished (middle trace), causing foreshortening of the bronchodilator response with 'rebound bronchospasm'

an analogous or identical mechanism, causes guinea-pigs to die when exposed to doses of airway spasmogens that would otherwise be innocuous. Since suppression of airway obstruction is the immediate consequence of exposure to rac-isoprenaline, sudden death would seem unlikely; however, following subcutaneous infusion of rac-isoprenaline (1 mg kg^{-1} day^{-1}) for 5 days, responsivity to inhaled allergen in sensitized guinea-pigs is increased such that animals invariably die soon after inhalation of allergen as during severe anaphylaxis (J. Morley, unpublished observations). These findings are consistent with earlier studies in which death occurred in response to lower doses of airway spasmogens following regular administration of rac-isoprenaline, rac-salbutamol or rac-terbutaline[15].

Inadvertently, we rediscovered this phenomenon whilst studying the capacity of rac-salbutamol and other antiasthma drugs to reduce airway eosinophilia in sensitized guinea-pigs, using a protocol in which antiasthma drugs (1 mg kg^{-1} day^{-1}) were administered subcutaneously over a 5-day period prior to inhalation of allergen[12]. Although infusion of rac-salbutamol by this route caused no obvious adverse effect in sensitized animals, exposure of such animals to inhaled allergen invariably resulted in severe dyspnoea and sudden death. Subsequent experiments revealed that this consequence of exposure to rac-salbutamol had become evident within 24 h and was lethal by 48 h. This effect of rac-salbutamol cannot be accounted for by adrenoceptor tachyphylaxis, since animals can be fully protected from the effects of inhaled allergen by subcutaneous injection of rac-salbutamol as a bolus (1 mg/kg) or by inhalation of rac-isoprenaline as an aerosol (10 μg/kg), immediately before inhalation of allergen.

By monitoring airway resistance and compliance in anaesthetized, sensitized animals before, during and after inhalation of allergen, it was possible to ascertain whether death might be attributed to acute airway obstruction. Bronchospasm which resulted from inhalation of allergen was heightened during prolonged exposure to rac-salbutamol, even though sensitivity to intravenous injection of histamine was slightly diminished[16]. This puzzling observation became intelligible when it was recognized that allergic airway hyper-reactivity is selective[17], so that acute airway obstruction in response to allergen is largely determined by rapid manifestation of increased responsivity to particular spasmogens, e.g. peptido-leukotrienes, platelet activating factor and kinins. It follows that development of airway hyper-reactivity due to rac-salbutamol might more readily be detected by use of such spasmogens. In guinea-pigs passively sensitized with antiserum 6 days prior to intravenous injection of a low dose of antigen, pronounced increased responsivity to intravenous injection of leukotriene C_4 results from exposure to antigen. In such animals, sustained infusion of rac-salbutamol (< 1 μg kg^{-1} min^{-1} for 5 days) induces increased responsivity to leukotriene C_4 prior to infusion of allergen; hence, animals can exhibit overt airway obstruction during infusion of allergen as well as developing enhanced hyper-reactivity of the airways thereafter[18]. When animals exhibit pronounced airway hyper-reactivity following subcutaneous infusion of rac-salbutamol, they have to be excluded from study of allergic reactions since death may antecede completion of the experimental protocol. To ascertain the possible involvement of enantiomers in this form of airway hyper-reactivity, sensitivity of normal animals to intravenous injection of leukotriene C_4 was defined before, and after, an infusion of (+)salbutamol (100 μg/kg over 1 h)[18]. The evident capacity of (+)salbutamol to evoke airway hyper-reactivity, and the resistance of this form of hyper-reactivity to rac-propranolol and susceptibility to vagal section, implies a mechanism similar to or identical with, that characterized for rac-isoprenaline[13].

AIRWAY HYPER-REACTIVITY IN COMPROMISED ANIMALS

Airway pharmacology of antiasthma drugs is typically defined using normal animals and sensitization to antigen is used solely to provide a more complex category of acute airway obstruction. However, expression of allergic reactions in guinea-pigs may modify responsivity of target cells qualitatively as well as quantitatively[19], raising the possibility that reactions to sympathomimetics may be influenced by immunological responses. Variation in the susceptibility of different batches of guinea-pigs to infused rac-isoprenaline was the first indication of this possibility and prompted study of animals subjected to antibody (immunoglobulin E)-mediated and cellular (Type IV hypersensitivity) immune reactions. Sensitization using an emulsion of antigen in alum together with injection of *Bordetella pertussis* is associated with preferential generation of immunoglobulin E and such animals exhibit heightened responsivity to platelet activating factor, which in the case of airway eosinophils can be presumed to be secondary to generation of cytokines[20]. Intratracheal instillation of small quantities (10 μg/animal) of (+)isoprenaline, (+)salbutamol or (+)terbutaline induced airway hyper-reactivity more effectively in animals sensitized in this way than in normal animals. Animals which have been sensitized using an emulsion of an antigen in Freund's complete adjuvant, exhibit selective reduction of dynamic compliance as a manifestation of cellular immunity without prominent airway hyper-reactivity 24 h after inhalation of antigen. In these circumstances, rac-isoprenaline more readily induces airway hyper-reactivity, though to what extent impaired compliance *per se* contributes to this effect has yet to be investigated.

Dying asthmatics may consume large quantities of sympathomimetics[21]. If the pharmacological processes defined for guinea-pigs extend to man, it should be recognized that loss of clinical benefit may depend not only on dosage and duration of sympathomimetic therapy, but also host reactions to

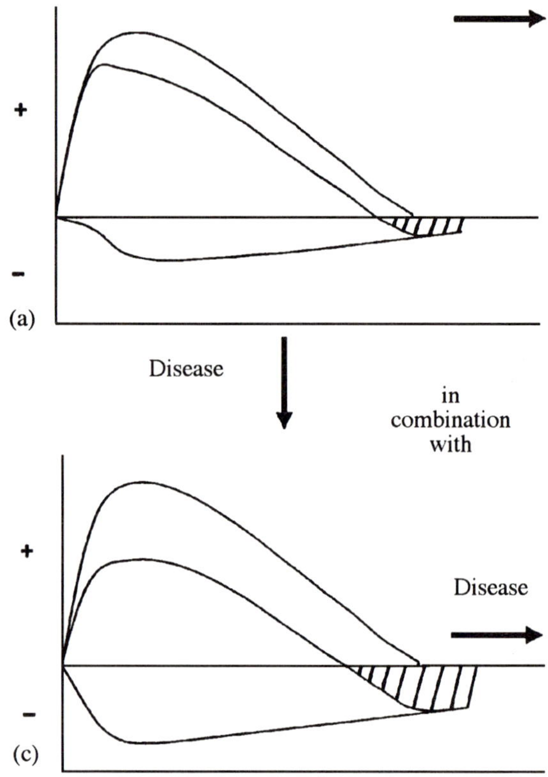

Figure 2 (a) Diagrammatic representation of effects of racemic sympathomimetics as described in Figure 1; (b) effect of repeated exposure to adrenoceptor stimulation, leading to diminished reduction of airway hyper-reactivity without change of the enhancement of airway hyper-reactivity due to the D-enantiomer; (c) maintained response to adrenoceptor activation follows acute allergic reaction of delayed hyper-reactivity together with an enhanced airway hyper-reactivity due

infection of inhaled noxae. It can be presumed that interaction between these unrelated processes will be additive and could thereby cause a precipitate transformation from net benefit to net deficit (Figure 2).

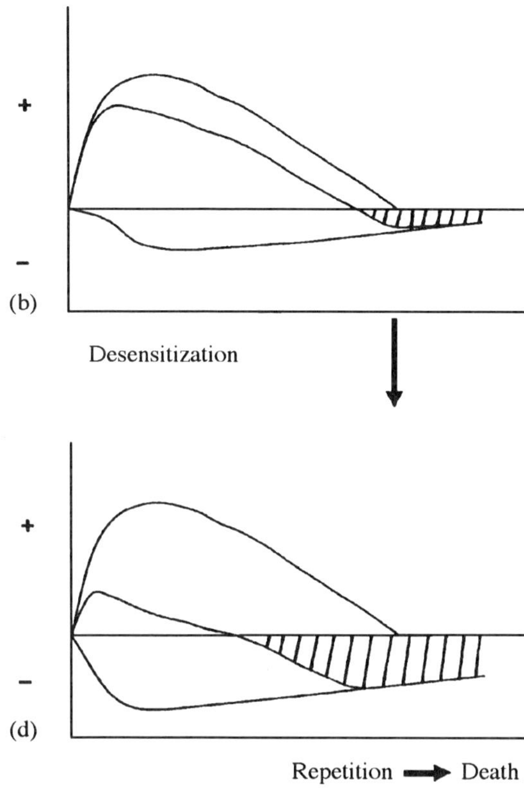

to the D-enantiomer; (d) reduced response to adrenoceptor stimulation coupled with enhanced airway hyper-reactivity due to the D-enantiomer causes profound suppression of the bronchodilator response and exaggeration of increased airway reactivity. Repeated dosing can be expected to convert the modest bronchodilator response (d) into a reaction in which *enhanced* airway reactivity predominates

DRUG EFFECTS

There is obvious interest in using drugs to pre-empt or reverse the adverse effects of sympathomimetics. In the guinea-pig, this form of airway hyper-reactivity is relatively difficult to inhibit if compared with hyper-reactivity due to allergen, immune complexes, endotoxin, or platelet activating factor. Of existing antiasthma therapies, only the effects of acute intraduodenal ketotifen and intraduodenal hydrocortisone have been studied in detail. Ketotifen (6 μg/kg intraduodenally) selectively and substantially (50%) inhibited the hyper-reactivity attributable to subcutaneous infusion of salbutamol (1 mg kg^{-1} day^{-1} for 6 days) in the guinea-pig, whereas larger doses (< 100 μg/kg) were needed to suppress to a comparable extent hyper-reactivity attributable to an acute allergic reaction. Substantially greater doses of hydrocortisone intraduodenally (> 1 mg/kg) were needed to effect significant inhibition of allergic airway hyper-reactivity and no selective inhibition of the reaction to rac-salbutamol could be detected[22]. These laboratory findings are consistent with the limited complementary clinical information presently available. Thus, diminished bronchodilator effects (i.e. induced airway hyper-reactivity) following exposure to a range of doses of rac-salbutamol were pre-empted by therapeutic doses of ketotifen[23] and development of airway hyper-reactivity during regular treatment with rac-fenoterol was not influenced by concurrent use of inhaled glucocorticoids[4]. Other drug categories can suppress the development of airway hyper-reactivity which follows infusion of rac-isoprenaline in the guinea-pig, including potassium channel openers[24] and phosphodiesterase isoenzyme inhibitors[25]. When evaluating such drugs clinically, more attention will have to be given to concurrent sympathomimetic usage than is conventional.

PHARMACOLOGICAL MECHANISM

It is not known how sympathomimetic racemates induce airway hyper-reactivity. Since both enantiomers of isoprenaline and of propranolol share this property, an uptake system such as that in the endothelial cells of pulmonary capillaries may be implicated, anticipating the failure of infused rac-adrenaline to induce airway hyper-reactivity[13], since pulmonary endothelial cells do not extract adrenaline from the circulation[26]. Operation of an uptake system would account for the latency and progression of this reaction as well as for the more marked effects of sustained infusion. Acute induction of airway hyper-reactivity by sympathomimetics reflects an effect upon airway nerves. The possibility has yet to be excluded that trophic effects of regular doses of sympathomimetics may explain the occurrence of an increased incidence of nerves in airway smooth muscle[27], and hence intractable airway hyper-reactivity.

CONCLUSION

At present, the pharmacology of sympathomimetics is insufficiently defined to allow those physicians specializing in asthma therapy to assess risk–benefit relationships with any certainty. It is instructive to consider why such a situation has arisen. Over the last 50 years, empirical selection of novel drug candidates by reference to effects upon animals which exhibit disease syndromes, or components thereof, has been progressively superseded by selection of compounds which influence clearly defined physiological control systems (e.g. receptors for hormones, neurotransmitters or autocoids) often using automated cellular or subcellular test systems. Thus, cloning of a receptor using techniques of molecular biology, designing a selective antagonist with the aid of computer technology and minimal testing on living tissues is now widely viewed as adequate for selection of novel drugs. Such 'molecular biology to bedside' philosophy relies heavily upon the results of preliminary clinical evaluation to provide evidence of efficacy that justifies development of the compound as a therapy and *inter alia* to detect acute adverse effects. This approach to drug discovery is more rapid and cost-effective than traditional methods, but by avoiding expensive and protracted animal pharmacology, it has transferred the risks of morbidity or mortality to the patient population.

In the case of sympathomimetics, subcellular mechanisms have been heavily promoted and whole animal pharmacology has become a subordinate annex, serving only to confirm the precepts of adrenoceptor occupancy. In this, as in other therapeutic areas, pharmacologists (preclinical and clinical) would do well to remember that all compounds provided by chemists, molecular biologists or cell biologists should be regarded with circumspection. Our knowledge of cellular interactions remains too sparse to allow prediction of whole animal pharmacology and toxicology from *in vitro* data and, for the foreseeable future, extensive whole animal pharmacology and toxicology remain the only reliable methods for anticipating and analysing adverse effects *prior to* clinical evaluation. Even after 5 years of investigation, it has not proved possible to demonstrate in our laboratories anomalous properties of sympathomimetics *in vitro*. Those seeking to minimize or even abolish animal experiments should be aware that, at present, it is not possible even *to conceive* how these unusual properties of sympathomimetics could have been detected, except by use of whole animal pharmacology. Discovery of potentially lethal properties during clinical pharmacology or therapeutics should not be accepted as a research strategy; rather, it must be consigned to the policy of last resort.

REFERENCES

1. Morley, J. (1991). New drug developments for asthma. In Morley, J. (ed.) *Preventive Therapy in Asthma*, pp. 254–73. (London: Academic Press)
2. Paterson, J. W., Courtenay Evans, R. J. and Prime, F. J. (1971). Selectivity of bronchodilator action of salbutamol in asthmatic patients. *Br. J. Dis. Chest*, **65**, 21–38
3. Kerrebijn, K. F., Van Essen-Zandvliet, E. M. and Neijens, H. J. (1987). Effect of long-term treatment with inhaled corticosteroids and beta-agonists on the bronchial responsiveness in children with asthma. *J. Allergy Clin. Immunol.*, **79**, 653–9
4. Sears, M. R., Taylor, D. R., Print, C. G., Lake, D. G., Li, Q., Flannery, E. M., Yates, D. M., Lucas, M. K. and Herbison, G. P. (1990). Regular inhaled beta-agonist treatment in bronchial asthma. *Lancet*, **336**, 1391–6
5. Ahrens, R. C., Harris, J. B., Milavetz, G., Annis, L. and Ries, R. (1987). Use of bronchial provocation with histamine to compare the pharmacodynamics of inhaled albuterol and metaproterenol in patients with asthma. *J. Allergy Clin. Immunol.*, **79**, 876–82
6. Spitzer, W. O., Suissa, S., Ernst, P., Horwitz, R. I., Habbick, B., Cockcroft, D., Boivin, J-F., McNutt, M., Buist, A. S. and Rebuck, A. S. (1992). The use of beta-agonists and the risk of death and near death from asthma. *N. Engl. J. Med.*, **326**, 501–6
7. Van Metre, T. E. Jr. (1969). Adverse effects of inhalation of excessive amounts of nebulized isoproterenol in status asthmaticus *J. Allergy Clin. Immunol.*, **43**, 101–113
8. Sears, M. R. (1991). Dose reduction of beta-agonists in asthma. *Lancet*, **338**, 1331–2
9. Mazzoni, L., Morley, J., Page, C. P. and Sanjar, S. (1985). Induction of hyperreactivity by platelet activating factor in the guinea-pig. *J. Physiol.*, **365**, 107P
10. Sanjar, S., Aoki, S., Kings, M. and Morley, J. (1989). Sensitisation to antigen or treatment with rh-GMCSF intensifies the eosinophilic response to PAF in the guinea-pig. *Am. Rev. Respir. Dis.*, **139**, 371A
11. Sanjar, S. and Morley, J. (1988). Airway hyperreactivity. *Lancet*, **2**, 160–1

12. Sanjar, S., Aoki, S., Kristersson, A., Smith, D. and Morley, J. (1990). Antigen challenge induces pulmonary airway eosinophil accumulation and airway hyperreactivity in sensitised guinea-pigs: the effect of anti-asthma drugs. *Br. J. Pharmacol.*, **99**, 679–86
13. Sanjar, S., Kristersson, A., Mazzoni, L., Morley, J. and Schaeublin, E. (1990). Increased airway reactivity in the guinea-pig follows exposure to intravenous isoprenaline. *J. Physiol.*, **425**, 43–54
14. Reisman, R. E. (1970). Asthma induced by adrenergic aerosols. *J. Allergy*, **46**, 162–77
15. Conolly, M. E., Davies, D. S., Dollery, C. T. and George, C. F. (1971). Resistance to beta-adrenoceptor stimulants (a possible explanation for the rise in asthma deaths). *Br. J. Pharmacol.*, **43**, 389–402
16. Chapman, I. D., Mazzoni, L. and Morley, J. (1990). An anomalous effect of salbutamol in sensitised guinea-pigs. *Br. J. Pharmacol.*, **99**, 66P
17. Morley, J., Hoshiko, K. Foster, A., Chapman, I. D., and Mazzoni, L. (1992). The selective nature of airway hyperreactivity. *J. Physiol.*, **446**, 117P
18. Morley, J., Chapman, I. D., Foster, A., Hoshiko, K. and Mazzoni, L. (1992). Effects of (+) and racemic salbutamol on airway responses in the guinea-pig. *Br. J. Pharmacol.*, **104**, 295P
19. Sanjar, S., Mazzoni, L., Schaueblin, E., Smith, D. and Morley, J. (1989). The effect of prophylactic anti-asthma drugs on PAF-induced airway hyperreactivity. *Jpn. J. Pharmacol.*, **51**, 151–60
20. Kings, M. A., Chapman, I. D., Kristersson, A., Sanjar, S. and Morley, J. (1990). Human recombinant lymphokines and cytokines induce pulmonary eosinophilia in the guinea pig which is inhibited by ketotifen and AH 21-132. *Int. Arch. Allergy Appl. Immunol.*, **297**, 354–61
21. Sears, M. R. and Rea, H. H. (1987). Patients at risk for dying of asthma: New Zealand experience. *J. Allergy Clin. Immunol.*, **80**, 477–81
22. Hoshiko, K., Kristersson, A. and Morley, J. (1992). Ketotifen inhibits exacerbation of allergic airway hyperreactivity by racemic-salbutamol in the guinea-pig. *J. Allergy Clin. Immunol.*, in press
23. Pauwels, R. and Van Der Straeten, M. (1988). Ketotifen prevents bronchial beta-adrenergic tachyphylaxis in normal humans. *J. Allergy Clin. Immunol.*, **81**, 674–80
24. Chapman, I. D., Kritersson, A., Mathelin, G., Schaeublin, E., Mazzoni, L., Boubekeur, K., Murphy, N. and Morley, J. (1992). Effects of a potassium channel opener (SDZ PCO 400) on guinea-pig and human pulmonary airways. *Br. J. Pharmacol.*, **106**, 423–9

25. Kristersson, A., Morley, J. and Schaeublin, E. (1988). Properties of AH21-132 that could contribute to prophylactic activity in asthma. *Br. J. Pharmacol.*, **93**, 53P
26. Vane, J. R. (1969). The release and fate of vaso-activity hormones in the circulation. *Br. J. Pharmacol.*, **35**, 209–42
27. Ollerenshaw, S., Jarvis, D., Woolcock, A., Sullivan, C. and Scheibner, T. (1989). Absence of immunoreactive vasoactive intestinal polypeptide in tissue from the lungs of patients with asthma. *N. Engl. J. Med.*, **320**, 1244–8

DISCUSSION

Dr M. Johnson (UK) Has it been possible to carry out similar experiments in species other than the guinea-pig? Is this a phenomenon that crosses species?

Dr J. Morley I have not pursued that personally, because we use guinea-pigs. According to the literature, anomalous effects of isoprenaline have been demonstrated in the dog. However, the observers tried to interpret their finding in terms of adrenoceptor occupancy. These data are published and I think we ought therefore to look at the dog.

Reference

Cho, Y. W., Aviado, D. M. and Lish, P. M. (1968). Efficacy of a new bronchodilator, soterenol, on experimental locked-lung syndrome in dogs. *J. Allergy Clin. Immunol.*, **42**, 36–48

5

The influence of β-agonists on airway inflammation in asthma

P. H. Howarth, J. A. Roberts, P. Bradding, A. E. Walls and S. T. Holgate

---

Although β-adrenoceptor agonists are widely used in asthma for their bronchodilator effect this may not be their sole mechanism of action in this disease. β-adrenoceptors have been localized within the respiratory tract to submucosal glands, vascular endothelium, ciliated epithelium, mast cells, clara cells, type II pneumocytes and cholinergic ganglia in addition to airway smooth muscle[1]. Receptor subtyping has identified that the influence of β-agonists at these sites is mediated by β_2-receptors with the exception of submucosal glands where β_1-receptor stimulation induces an increase in glandular secretion.

Of relevance to the regulation of airway inflammation in asthma is the potential action of β_2-receptor stimulation on the vascular endothelium, ciliated epithelium and mast cells.

Mediators such as histamine, bradykinin, prostaglandins and leukotrienes, released from activated mast cells and eosinophils, interact with specific receptors located on the vascular endothelium of postcapillary vessels to induce contraction and the opening of gap junctions between adjacent cells[2,3]. This action will promote plasma protein extravasation and the development of mucosal oedema. This pro-inflammatory action is inhibited by prior administration of β-agonists[2]. A direct inhibitory effect of β_2-adrenoceptor stimulation on protein transit through an endothelial cell monolayer in asthma has been demonstrated *in vitro*[4]. Should such an action occur *in vivo* with prolonged β_2-adrenoceptor stimulation then not only would mucosal oedema be modified but the egression of cells through the vascular endothelium would also be reduced, as inflammatory cells di-apedese through gap junctions to obtain access to tissue sites. In addition to this direct effect, β-adrenoceptor stimulation may also indirectly influence changes in vascular permeability by modifying epithelial cell and mast cell function. β_2-receptor activation promotes tight junction binding between epithelial cells and may thus, in allergic asthma, reduce access of allergen to structures deep in the epithelium and thereby limit the allergic response[5]. Furthermore, it has long been recognized that β_2-agonists modulate immunoglobulin E-dependent mediator release from chopped human lung[6] and more detailed studies on dispersed human lung mast cells have suggested that salbutamol is 30 000 times as potent as sodium cromoglycate in inhibiting immunological mast cell degranulation[7].

Evidence has been obtained from indirect measurements that these non-bronchodilator actions of β-adrenoceptor stimulation occur *in vivo* in asthma with acute administration. Both salbutamol and terbutaline have been found to inhibit the increase in markers of mast cell activation in peripheral blood following allergen challenge[8,9] and both salmeterol and formoterol have been demonstrated to inhibit allergen-induced late-phase bronchoconstriction and acquisition of bronchial responsiveness, a response clinically associated with eosinophil influx and plasma protein extravasation[10,11]. To assess whether these actions occur in clinical disease with chronic therapy we have undertaken a detailed assessment of cell infiltration and cell activation within the airways *in vivo* in asthma, by fibre-optic bronchoscopy with endobronchial lavage and biopsy, before and after regular therapy with the potent, long-acting β-agonist, salmeterol.

Twenty-six atopic asthmatics whose sole therapy was an inhaled β-agonist on a *pro re nata* basis participated in the study. During a 2-week run-in period prior to the first bronchoscopy each patient recorded daily, in diary cards, their symptoms, peak flow (a.m. and p.m.) and their use of salbutamol on an as required basis. In addition each patient underwent methacholine inhalation challenge to determine their level of bronchial responsiveness, as identified by the provocative concentration required to produce a 20% fall in forced expiratory volume (FEV_1) (PC_{20}). All subjects had daily symptoms and hyper-reactive airways. Following the first bronchoscopy patients were randomly allocated to receive either inhaled salmeterol 50 μg twice a day ($n = 14$) or matched placebo ($n = 12$). This treatment, along with salbutamol on an as required basis, was continued for a 6-week period up to a second bronchoscopy. During this period patients continued their daily diary card recording. Each bronchoscopy was performed according to safety guidelines[12] and both endobronchial lavage and biopsy samples were obtained. The lavage was processed for total cell count, differential cell count,

T-lymphocyte subset and activation status by flow cytometry, and measurement of supernatant levels of histamine, tryptase, eosinophil cationic protein and albumin. The bronchial biopsies were processed into methacrylate resin for immunohistochemical staining with monoclonal antibodies directed against mast cells (AAI – antitryptase) eosinophils (EG2 – anti-eosinophil cationic protein) and T lymphocytes (CD3, CD4, CD8). The presence of immunostaining was revealed by using the streptoavidin–biotin–peroxidase system with aminoethylcarbazone as the detection system. The number of positively staining cells with each antibody was counted in five adjacent sections 10 μm apart and the results were expressed for the submucosa in relation to the area assessed (cells/mm^2).

Twenty-three patients completed the study, salmeterol ($n = 12$), placebo ($n = 11$). Only one of the three drop-outs was related to disease exacerbation (placebo). Regular salmeterol therapy was associated with symptomatic improvement ($p < 0.001$) and a mean increase in peak flow a.m. (68 l/min, $p < 0.001$) and p.m. (59 l/min, $p < 0.01$). The PC_{20} values did not change with placebo therapy but were physiologically displaced in the salmeterol group during therapy ($p < 0.03$), rising from 0.5 mg/ml to 1.9 mg/ml. Analysis of both lavage and biopsy results from salmeterol- and placebo-treated groups revealed no difference between the before and 6-week findings[13,14].

Thus, this study has not found evidence that regular β-agonist therapy in chronic disease alters the airway inflammatory profile when numbers of mast cells, eosinophils and T lymphocytes are assessed in biopsies and these cell populations plus macrophages are analysed in lavage. Furthermore, analysis of histamine, tryptase and eosinophil cationic protein levels in lavage and the cell surface expression of CD25 (interleukin-2 receptor) and human leukocyte antigen locus DR on CD3 positive T lymphocytes was unchanged, indicating that the state of cell activation, which is increased in asthma[15], was also unaltered. There was no resolution or deterioration in these findings. This would suggest that the clinical and physiological improvement seen with regular therapy relates to the bronchodilator properties of β-receptor stimulation rather than the non-bronchodilator effects. This finding has important implications with respect both to the understanding of acute and chronic airway inflammation and to the positioning of β-agonists in the management of asthma.

Firstly, these findings with regular therapy in chronic disease differ from single dose administration in acute induced disease, both in the airways[8–10] and in the skin[16]. Within the skin, intradermal application of a β-agonist prior to intradermal allergen reduced both the early and late responses[16] and the late accumulation of eosinophils[17]. Similarly, in an animal model of asthma, salmeterol has been shown to prevent the late increase in lung eosinophils following allergen challenge[18]. These acute responses do, however, relate to high allergen loads and the response is mast cell-dependent[19], whereas the T lymphocyte has been emphasized as an orchestrator of cell influx in chronic disease[20]. While these considerations suggest a difference between acute and chronic inflammation, this alone cannot explain the lack of effect of salmeterol in this study as no influence could be detected on mast cell histamine and tryptase levels in lavage. This contrasts with previous *in vitro* studies with lung mast cells[6,7]. As mast cell inhibition is dose-dependent[7] it is possible that at 50 μg twice a day there is insufficient local concentration of salmeterol on luminal mast cells to inhibit degranulation, but sufficient to relax airway smooth muscle. This requires further evaluation. Secondly, this study does not identify any deterioration in either symptoms, bronchial responsiveness or airway inflammation with salmeterol therapy and over the 6-week period of treatment no data have been found to support the concepts that regular β-agonist therapy makes asthma worse[21] and that this is due to an inhibitory effect on airway mast cells[22]. The findings of a lack of effect on inflammatory indices in contrast to the influence of corticosteroid therapy in a similar investigation[23] does, however, reinforce the recently published guidelines on asthma management[24] which advocates the use of short-term β-agonists only on a *pro re nata* basis with the early introduction of inhaled prophylactic anti-inflammatory therapy in patients with daily symptoms. The present findings suggest that the long-acting β-agonists cannot act as a substitute for currently accepted inhaled prophylactic anti-inflammatory therapies and that their use should be in patients receiving such therapy who remain symptomatic.

REFERENCES

1. Barnes, P. J. (1984). Beta-adrenoceptors in lung tissue. In Marley, J. (ed.) *Beta-adrenoceptors in Asthma*, pp. 67–90. (London: Academic Press)
2. Persson, C. G. A., Ergefalt, I., Grega, C. I. and Svensjo, E. (1982). The role of β-receptor agonists in the inhibition of pulmonary oedema. *Ann. N. Y. Acad. Sci.*, **384**, 544–56

3. Minnear, F. L., DeMichele, M. A., Moon, D. S., Reider, C. L. and Fenton, J. W. (1989). Isoproterenol reduces thrombin induced pulmonary endothelial permeability *in vitro*. *Am. J. Physiol.*, **257**, H1613–23
4. Gudgeon, J. R. and Martin, W. (1989). Modulation of arterial endothelial permeability: studies on an *in vitro* model. *Br. J. Pharmacol.*, **98**, 1267–74
5. Duffy, M. E., Hainan, B., Hos, S. and Bentgel, C. J. (1981). Regulation of epithelial tight junction permeability by cyclic AMP. *Nature (London)*, **294**, 451–3
6. Assem, E. S. K. and Schild, H. O. (1989). Inhibition of sympathomimetic amines of histamine release induced by antigen in passively sensitised human lung. *Nature (London)*, **224**, 1028–9
7. Church, M. K., Holgate, S. T. and Pao, G. J. K. (1983). Histamine release from mechanically and enzymatically dispersed human lung mast cells: inhibition by salbutamol and cromoglycate. *Br. J. Pharmacol.*, **79** (Suppl.), 374P
8. Martin, G. L., Atkins, P. C., Dunsky, E. H. and Sweiman, B. (1980). Effects of theophylline, terbutaline and prednisolone on antigen-induced bronchospasm and mediator release. *J. Allergy Clin. Immunol.*, **66**, 204–12
9. Howarth, P. H., Durham, S. R., Lee, T. H., Kay, A. B., Church, M. K. and Holgate, S. T. (1985). Influence of albuterol, cromolyn sodium and ipratropium bromide on the airway and circulating mediator responses to allergen bronchial provocation in asthma. *Am. Rev. Respir. Dis.*, **132**, 986–92
10. Twentyman, O. P., Finnerty, J. P., Harris, A., Palmer, S. and Holgate, S. T. (1990). Protection against allergen-induced asthma by salmeterol. *Lancet*, **336**, 1338–42
11. Palmqvist, M., Lowhagen, O., Balder, B., Melander, B., Svedmyr, N. and Wahlander, L. (1991). Prevention of late asthmatic reaction by salbutamol and formoterol. *Eur. Respir. J.*, **8**, 768
12. Djukanovic, R., Wilson, J. W., Lai, C. K. W., Holgate, S. T. and Howarth, P. H. (1991). The safety aspects of fibreoptic bronchoscopy, bronchoalveolar lavage and endobronchial biopsy in asthma. *Am. Rev. Respir. Dis.*, **143**, 772–7
13. Roberts, J. A., Bradding, P., Walls, A. F., Britten, K. M., Wilson, S., Holgate, S. T. and Howarth, P. H. (1992). The influence of by salmeterol xinafoate on mucosal inflammation in asthma. *Am. Rev. Respir. Dis.*, **145**, A418
14. Roberts, J. A., Bradding, P., Walls, A. F., Holgate, S. T. and Howarth, P. H. (1992). The effect of salmeterol xinafoate therapy on lavage findings in asthma. *Am. Rev. Respir. Dis.*, **145**, A418
15. Howarth, P. H., Wilson, J., Djukanovic, R., Wilson, S., Britten, K., Walls, A., Roche, W. R. and Holgate, S. T. (1991). Airway inflammation and atopic

asthma: a comparative bronchoscopic investigation. *Int. Arch. Allergy Appl. Immunol.*, **14**, 266–9

16. Gronneberg, R. and Zetterstrom, O. (1990). Inhibition of anti-IgE induced skin response in normals by formoterol, a new β_2-adrenoceptor agonist, and terbutaline. 2. Effect on late phase reactions. *Allergy*, **45**, 340–6
17. Ting, S., Zweiman, B. and Larker, R. (1983). Terbutaline modulation of human allergic skin reactions. *J. Allergy Clin. Immunol.*, **71**, 437–41
18. Sanjar, S., McCabe, P. J. and Humbles, A. H. (1991). Inhibition by salmeterol of antigen-induced eosinophil accumulation in guinea-pig lung. *Environ. Res. J.*, **4**, 200S
19. Howarth, P. H., Durham, S. R., Kay, A. B. and Holgate, S. T. (1987). The relationship between mast cell mediator release and bronchial reactivity in allergic asthma. *J. Allergy Clin. Immunol.*, **80**, 703–11
20. Corrigan, C. J. and Kay, A. B. (1990). CD4 T-lymphocyte activation in acute severe asthma: relationship to disease severity and atopic status. *Am. Rev. Respir. Dis.*, **141**, 970–7
21. Sears, M. R., Taylor, D. R., Print, C. G., Lake, D. C., Li, Q. and Flannery, E. M. (1990). Regular inhaled beta-agonist treatment of bronchial asthma. *Lancet*, **336**, 1391–6
22. Page, C. (1991). One explanation of the asthma paradox: inhibition of natural anti-inflammatory mechanism by β_2-agonists. *Lancet*, **337**, 717–20
23. Djukanovic, R., Wilson, J. W., Britten, K. M., Wilson, S. J., Walls, A. F., Roche, W. R., Howarth, P. H. and Holgate, S. T. (1992). The effect of an inhaled corticosteroid on airway inflammation and symptoms in asthma. *Am. Rev. Respir. Dis.*, **145**, 669–74
24. Guidelines for management of asthma in adults: I. Chronic persistent asthma. *Br. Med. J.*, **301**, 651–3

DISCUSSION

Dr H. Smith (Smith Kline Beecham) You have shown that salmeterol has no effect on chronic inflammation in the airways. It is assumed that steroids would do this. Do you know if any equally careful study has been carried out to prove that steroids really do what everyone thinks they do?

Dr P. H. Howarth This is not my remit today, but we have carried out similar studies with inhaled beclomethasone and showed that this reduces the eosinophil populations in the airways, reduces the epithelial and lavage mast cell numbers – which is coincidental with the reduction in tryptase and histamine levels – and decreases the T lymphocyte activation status to normal. It has therefore been possible to demonstrate in a separate study that these effects can be identified.

Chairman's summary

S. T. Holgate

I hope everybody agrees that it has been a most stimulating session. We have heard about a range of interesting new methodologies being applied to studying the potential role of β-agonists in bronchial asthma.

Prof. Barnes focused our minds very much on the molecular biological aspects of the β-receptor, and introduced some quite interesting ideas about what may be happening in relation to up- and down-regulation of receptor function. He also touched on the possibility of there being more than two β-receptor subtypes. Clearly, with the exploration of the human genome, it is likely that more will be found out about these various types of β-receptor.

Dr Johnson took up an issue that Prof. Barnes started with, the interaction of the β-agonist with its receptor and the sites of binding within the membrane domains. He illustrated how he felt salmeterol and formoterol may be binding as a new class of β-agonists to within the β-receptor domain in a rather unusual fashion involving, first, solution in the lipid bilayer and then binding to a site adjacent to, but distant from, the G-protein activation site of the β-receptor.

Using rather elegant pharmacological techniques in animals, he then illustrated how both formoterol and salmeterol could be explained in terms of their pharmacology on the basis of this somewhat unusual binding characteristic.

Finally, he drew our attention to the fact that β-agonists have effects other than relaxing the smooth muscle. He focused on the availability of these drugs to inhibit both microvascular permeability and eosinophil migration into the guinea-pig lung following allergen challenge, and also to have effects – so far not too well documented – on macrophages and cilial beat frequency.

This class of compounds clearly has interesting effects outside of smooth muscle. As Prof. Barnes raised during his presentation, β-receptors are found in many other sites in the airway than in smooth muscle, including the alveoli and mucous glands, that we have yet to learn much about in terms of mechanism.

Dr Page picked up the interesting idea that the mast cell may be a protective cell in the airway, which has evolved phylogenetically to protect against inhaled substances, especially allergens. From his review of the literature in a number of different areas, he presented an interesting case for a protective role in particular for the glycosaminoglycans and heparin specifically. He also talked about the possible effect of these proteoglycans in suppressing some of the T cell-mediated functions of our immune system. As we have heard already, the T-cell seems to be assuming an important role in asthma.

It remains to be seen whether or not this hypothesis will stand the test of time and it depends on people like Dr Page and others to challenge it with experiments in humans and animals to see whether his work can be substantiated.

Dr Morley reported some of his animal experiments, focusing very much on the guinea-pig, on hyper-reactivity provoked by platelet activating factor and other mediators. He presented a case for hyper-reactivity being a heterogeneous response in the guinea-pig airway, and for one of these heterogeneous responses being induced by prior treatment of animals with β-agonists. He argued that this was not a β_2-receptor-mediated effect, nor indeed did he think it was a β-receptor-mediated effect at all but probably involves the stimulation of afferent neurons and neural reflexes. He went on to say that this may in fact relate in some way to the adverse effects of β-agonists in asthma. He described some studies that he and his colleagues have done with racemic mixtures of β-agonists and the separate enantiomers, arguing that the S enantiomer in particular, of a number of β-agonists in this particular model, was active in enhancing reactivity to a number of different agents.

Finally, Dr Howarth brought us back to the human question, and very much the chronicity of the inflammatory response in a single clinical trial involving 6 weeks of treatment with regular β-agonists. He demonstrated that in the face of good clinical response as far as the patients were concerned, he was not able to demonstrate from a number of different measurements a change either in the inflammatory cells or in their mediators within the airway.

I think, therefore, that a large number of important biomedical issues still need to be addressed in looking at the role of β-agonists in asthma. It is my view – and I am sure everybody else's – that this field is far from being completely worked out.

6

Should we be using β-agonists for treatment of chronic asthma?

M. R. Sears

A number of studies have raised the question of how β-agonists should be used in the management of bronchial asthma. In addressing this topic, I will discuss the use of currently available short-acting β-agonists, and leave long-acting β-agonists to be discussed elsewhere in this volume.

Inhaled short-acting β-agonists have been used for several decades in relieving symptoms of asthma, and have an essential role in providing rapid relief of the dyspnoea, wheezing and coughing associated with acute asthma[1]. Even when asthmatics have used a considerable amount of inhaled β-agonist prior to presenting to an Emergency Room, effective bronchodilatation can be achieved with the use of high doses[2]. However, the efficacy of inhaled bronchodilator in treating acute asthma may be limited, and full reversal of airway narrowing is seldom achieved unless the attack is mild. Failure to achieve full reversal is more likely to relate to the severity of airflow obstruction due to mucosal oedema and secretions, than to tachyphylaxis to the inhaled β-agonist[3].

A major concern has been raised about chronic use of inhaled short-acting β-agonists to maintain bronchodilatation or prevent bronchoconstriction. While as yet only one specifically designed study has clearly demonstrated an adverse effect of regular β-agonist therapy[4], evidence is accumulating to suggest that regular use of inhaled short-acting β-agonists may impair the long-term control of asthma as judged by symptoms, lung function and measurements of airway responsiveness[5–16].

A randomized, double-blind, placebo-controlled, cross-over study undertaken in New Zealand (1988–90), was recently reported, in which subjects inhaled dry powder fenoterol 400 μg four times a day or matching placebo for 6 months, then crossed to the alternative regime[4]. Throughout the entire study, subjects used an additional known bronchodilator for relief of symptoms when required. Subjects were maintained on inhaled corticosteroid in the dose taken prior to entry to the study, but theophylline, ipratropium and oral β-agonists were prohibited. Subjects, who were provided with a new bottle of dry powder capsules every 4 weeks, were unaware of the study design or that only one active agent was used. Subjects recorded morning and evening peak flow rates, nocturnal and daytime symptoms, use of additional inhaled β-agonist, and use of short courses of prednisone. The period of better control of asthma was determined in each subject by comparing the final 16 weeks of each treatment period (an 8-week washout period was excluded from the beginning of each period). Statistically significant differences in each of seven markers of control were used to ascertain whether the subject was better controlled in the first or second treatment period. Of 64 patients completing this study, 57 showed better control in one or other period; 40 of these 57 (70%) showed better control when β-agonist was inhaled only when needed, i.e. had worse control of asthma when inhaled β-agonists were taken regularly. This difference was most clearly reflected in the morning peak flow rates, but other markers of control also showed preferences for the placebo period; the one exception was the evening peak flow rate which, being measured 3–4 h following the last dose of inhaled bronchodilator, was generally higher during the period of active therapy.

An unexpected finding from this study was that the deleterious effects of regular inhaled β-agonists were not obviated by the use of any dose of inhaled corticosteroid. Even subjects taking more than 800 μg inhaled corticosteroid daily showed the same trend towards worsening asthma when using regular inhaled β-agonist. Of eight patients using 1500 μg inhaled corticosteroid or more daily, seven became worse with regular inhaled β-agonist and improved when β-agonist was used only as required for control of symptoms.

The occurrence of an exacerbation was determined by the simultaneous appearance of two or more predefined criteria. Exacerbations occurred earlier and more frequently during regular therapy. There were significant differences in the number of subjects who had experienced an exacerbation after 1 month and 2 months of each treatment regimen; fewer subjects had exacerbations when using bronchodilator only as needed. Six severe exacerbations occurred during the study, five requiring hospitalization and one requiring the patient to temporarily withdraw from the study; five of these

Table 1 Effects of regular inhaled or oral β-agonist on lung function in asthmatics

Drug	*Duration* (weeks)	*Variable*★	*Baseline value*	*Regular treatment*	*p*	*Reference*
Fenoterol	24	FEV_1	2.46	2.29	< 0.05	4
Salbutamol	4	FEV_1	2.30	2.08	NS	6
Salbutamol	4	FEV_1	3.68	3.33	< 0.05	8
Fenoterol	4	FEV_1	2.76	2.43	< 0.05	10
Fenoterol (Oral)	12	FEV_1	2.53	2.05	< 0.05	11
Ephedrine (Oral)	12	FEV_1	2.25	2.08	< 0.05	11

★FEV_1, forced expiratory volume in one second (l); NS = not significant

Table 2 Effects of regular β-agonist on airway responsiveness (PC_{20} (mg/ml) or PD_{20} (μg) to histamine or methacholine

Drug	*Duration* (weeks)	*Variable*★	*Baseline value*	*Regular treatment*	*p*†	*Reference*
Fenoterol	24	PC_{20}	1.53	1.03	< 0.05	4
Terbutaline	2	PC_{20}	4.7	3.1	< 0.01	12
Terbutaline	26	PD_{20}	43	27	NR	13
Salbutamol	52	PC_{20}	13.2	7.9	< 0.005	14
Salbutamol	4	PC_{20}	1.16	0.74	NR	15

★PC_{20}, provocative concentration required to cause 20% drop in forced expiratory volume; PD_{20}, provocative dose required to cause 20% drop in forced expiratory volume; NR = †not reported

six severe exacerbations occurred when the subject was taking regular β-agonist.

A number of studies suggest that lung function may be impaired by the regular use of different inhaled β-agonists (Table 1). Similarly, several studies have shown adverse effects of regular inhaled β-agonists on airway hyper-responsiveness (Table 2). It therefore seems unlikely that these adverse effects are drug specific, but rather represent a class effect of inhaled short-acting β-agonists. The adverse effect of fenoterol (a more potent bronchodilator which was marketed at a higher dose per puff) is probably more striking than has been previously seen with other inhaled β-agonists, thus accounting for the fact that until our study was published, these other findings had been largely overlooked.

The finding that regular inhaled β-agonist therapy is deleterious in asthma provides an explanation for the increasing morbidity and mortality from asthma over recent decades, and for the two major epidemics of asthma mortality[17,18]. Our study has shown that mild asthma can be converted into moderate asthma and even into severe asthma by the use of regular inhaled β-agonist therapy, the primary treatment offered to new mild and moderate asthmatics. It is therefore conceivable that we have unknowingly changed the severity of the disease by using what appeared to be effective short-term therapy. Once asthma has become severe, the use of further doses of inhaled β-agonist, often given on a regular schedule in high doses including nebulized therapy, contributes to increasing morbidity. Hence, a vicious circle is set up whereby severe asthma is treated with more bronchodilator thus increasing further the severity of asthma. The use of inhaled (and probably of oral) corticosteroids, while beneficial to many patients with chronic severe asthma, does not obviate the adverse effect of regular inhaled β-agonist, and so patients remain in this vicious circle despite high-dose steroid therapy. Once severe asthma has developed, the stage is set for hospital admissions and for fatal episodes, which may occur when the patient is inadequately or inappropriately treated for a severe attack of asthma. While we now know a great deal about the circumstances of fatal attacks, studies of fatal asthma have not adequately explained why asthma was of such severity as to put the patient at risk of a fatal episode. The hypothesis we have developed relating to an increase in the chronic severity of asthma induced by the frequent use of inhaled β-agonist does explain this increase in severity.

A number of critics have drawn attention to other studies purportedly showing that regular β-agonist therapy is beneficial in asthma[5,19–22]. Space does not permit review of all of these studies, but all have major inadequacies which preclude their use to support regular β-agonist therapy. Two studies from the United Kingdom will serve to illustrate the erroneous conclusions drawn from these studies. Shepherd and colleagues[19] conducted a very short cross-over study in 18 subjects, with 1 week of each treatment, comparing salbutamol, two puffs four times a day, with salbutamol, strictly *pro re nata*. The only statistically significant finding in this study was that the evening peak flow rate improved on regular salbutamol therapy, a finding exactly mirrored in our own study[4]. All other findings were not statistically significant. The short duration of this study means that any long-term adverse effects were not seen. A much longer study using a parallel group design followed by a cross-over period was reported by Beswick and colleagues[5]. Their subjects were given salbutamol or placebo, two puffs four times a day, regularly for 1 year; each group had access to intermittent β-agonist as needed for symptoms. After 12 months, the groups crossed over to the alternative regimen for 3 months. The authors reported stable peak flow rates during 12 months of treatment with regular salbutamol, whereas those using salbutamol only as needed, showed 'unstable' peak flow rates. However, when mean peak flow rates are plotted by time, it is evident that the 'instability' reflected improving peak flow rates, especially during the latter 6 months of the treatment period. When these patients then used regular therapy, peak flow declined to less than the baseline value. Rather than showing the beneficial effects of regular therapy in maintaining stability of peak flow, this study supports our conclusion that regular β-agonist is deleterious to pulmonary function.

When β-agonist therapy is used on a strictly as needed basis, the number of puffs required each day is a useful marker of the degree of control of asthma, and the adequacy of alternative non-bronchodilator therapy. Such a marker is lost when β-agonist is given on a regular scheduled basis. There is some evidence that regular bronchodilator therapy can cause minor tachyphylaxis, as seen in our study, but we have found that bronchodilator taken only when needed is more effective than when used in conjunction with regular therapy. Use of β-agonist therapy only as needed may also improve compliance with anti-inflammatory therapy.

Further evidence against the regular use of inhaled β-agonist therapy has come from clinical studies of the effect of withdrawing high-dose or frequently inhaled β-agonist in patients with moderate to severe asthma. If our hypothesis that regular use of β-agonist therapy may increase the severity of asthma is correct, the logical corollary is that reduction in β-agonist use may reverse this process. We have observed this in many subjects, confirming observations made over 20 years ago when isoprenaline was used in the management of asthma[23–26]. The subject with unstable asthma who apparently needs regular doses of inhaled bronchodilator frequently becomes more stable when bronchodilator use is minimized. This effect is seen in children and adults irrespective of the drug used, and has been seen in subjects with apparently severe irreversible asthma, in whom the severity of obstruction has declined as β-agonists have been withdrawn.

A simple, effective protocol for reduction of inhaled β-agonist has recently been published[27]. Briefly, peak flow rates are monitored for 7–14 days while baseline therapy is continued. Then, without changing any other therapy, the patient is asked to use an inhaled bronchodilator only if the peak flow falls below a certain level, which is generally set at about 50% of the best achieved peak flow. Improvements in peak flow can be seen as early as a few days after this change, but some patients take several weeks to show the increased lung function and reduction in symptoms which has occurred in virtually every case where this strategy has been applied.

In summary, there is a place for using inhaled short-acting β-agonists in the treatment of asthma, namely their use in reversing acute episodes which break through maintenance therapy with anti-inflammatory and anti-allergic medication in combination with avoidance measures. There is, however, no place for the use of short-acting β-agonists on a regularly scheduled basis for control of asthma, as there is considerable evidence to suggest that in the long-term such treatment is deleterious to the control of asthma.

REFERENCES

1. Price, A. H. and Clissold, S. P. (1989). Salbutamol in the 1980's. A reappraisal of its clinical efficacy. *Drugs*, **38**, 77–122
2. Rossing, T. H., Fanta, C. H. and McFadden, E. R. (1983). Effect of outpatient treatment of asthma with beta agonists on the response to sympathomimetics in an emergency room. *Am. J. Med.*, **75**, 781–4
3. Sheffer, A. L. and Fink, J. N. (1991). Asthma '90. Immunopharmacological update. *J. Allergy Clin. Immunol.*, **88**, 303–21
4. Sears, M. R., Taylor, D. R., Print, C. G., Lake, D. C., Li, Q., Flannery, E. M., Yates, D. M., Lucas, M. K. and Herbison, G. P. (1990). Regular inhaled beta-agonist treatment in bronchial asthma. *Lancet*, **336**, 1391–6
5. Beswick, K. B. J., Pover, G. M. and Sampson, S. (1986). Long-term regularly inhaled salbutamol. *Curr. Med. Res. Opin.*, **10**, 228–34
6. Patakas, D., Maniki, E., Tsara, V. and Daskalopoulou, E. (1988). Intermittent and continuous salbutamol rotacaps inhalation in asthmatic patients. *Respiration*, **54**, 174–8
7. van Schayck, C. P., Dompeling, E., van Herwaarden, C. L. A., Folgering, H., Verbeek, A. L. M., van der Hoogen, H. J. M. and van Weel, C. (1991). Bronchodilator treatment in moderate asthma or chronic bronchitis: continuous or on demand? A randomised controlled study. *Br. Med. J.*, **303**, 1426–31

8. Harvey, J. E. and Tattersfield, A. E. (1982). Airway response to salbutamol: effect of regular salbutamol inhalations in normal, atopic, and asthmatic subjects. *Thorax*, **37**, 280–7
9. Gibson, G. J., Greenacre, J. K., Konig, P., Conolly, M. E. and Pride, N. B. (1978). Use of exercise challenge to investigate possible tolerance to beta-adrenoceptor stimulation in asthma. *Br. J. Dis. Chest*, **72**, 199–206
10. Trembath, P. W., Greenacre, J. K., Anderson, M., Dimmock, S., Mansfield, L., Wadsworth, J. and Green, M. (1979). Comparison of four weeks' treatment with fenoterol and terbutaline aerosols in adult asthmatics. A double-blind crossover study. *J. Allergy Clin. Immunol.*, **63**, 395–400
11. VanArsdel, P. P., Schaffrin, R. M., Rosenblatt, J., Sprenkle, A. C. and Altman, L. C. (1978). Evaluation of oral fenoterol in chronic asthmatic patients. *Chest*, **73**, 997–8
12. Kraan, J., Koeter, G. H., v.d.Mark, Th. W., Sluiter, H. J. and de Vries, K. (1985). Changes in bronchial hyperreactivity induced by 4 weeks of treatment with antiasthmatic drugs in patients with allergic asthma: a comparison between budesonide and terbutaline. *J. Allergy Clin. Immunol.*, **76**, 628–36
13. Kerrebijn, K. F., van Essen-Zandvliet, E. E. M. and Neijens, H. J. (1987). Effect of long-term treatment with inhaled corticosteroids and beta-agonists on the bronchial responsiveness in children with asthma. *J. Allergy Clin. Immunol.*, **79**, 653–9
14. van Schayck, C. P., Graafsma, S. J., Visch, M. B., Dompeling, E., van Weel, C. and van Herwaarden, C. L. A. (1990). Increased bronchial hyperresponsiveness after inhaling salbutamol during 1 year is not caused by sensitization to salbutamol. *J. Allergy Clin. Immunol.*, **86**, 793–800
15. Peel, E. T. and Gibson, G. J. (1980). Effects of long-term inhaled salbutamol therapy on the provocation of asthma by histamine. *Am. Rev. Respir. Dis.*, **121**, 973–8
16. Vathenen, A. S., Knox, A. J., Higgins, B. G., Britton, J. R. and Tattersfield, A. E. (1988). Rebound increase in bronchial responsiveness after treatment with inhaled terbutaline. *Lancet*, **1**, 554–8
17. Stolley, P. D. and Schinnar, R. (1978). Association between asthma mortality and isoproterenol aerosols: a review. *Prevent. Med.*, **7**, 519–38
18. Grainger, J., Woodman, K., Pearce, N., Crane, J., Burgess, C., Keane, A. and Beasley, R., (1991). Prescribed fenoterol and death from asthma in New Zealand, 1981–7: a further case–control study. *Thorax*, **46**, 105–11

19. Shepherd, G. L., Hetzel, M. R. and Clark, T. J. H. (1981). Regular versus symptomatic aerosol bronchodilator treatment of asthma. *Br. J. Dis. Chest*, **75**, 215–17
20. Vandewalker, M. L., Kray, K. T., Weber, R. W. and Nelson, H. S. (1986). Addition of terbutaline to optimal theophylline therapy. Double blind cross-over study in asthmatic patients. *Chest*, **90**, 198–203
21. Smith, J. A., Weber, R. W. and Nelson, H. S. (1980). Theophylline and aerosolized terbutaline in the treatment of bronchial asthma. Double-blind comparison of optimal doses. *Chest*, **78**, 816–18
22. Shepherd, G. L., Jenkins, W. J. and Alexander, J. (1991). Asthma exacerbations in patients taking regular salmeterol, or salbutamol for symptoms. *Lancet*, **337**, 1424
23. Keighley, J. F. (1966). Iatrogenic asthma associated with adrenergic aerosols. *Ann. Int. Med.*, **65**, 985–95
24. Eisenstadt, W. S. and Nicholas, S. S. (1969). The adverse effect of adrenergic aerosols in bronchial asthma. *Ann. Allergy*, **27**, 283–8
25. Van Metre, T. E., Jr. (1969). Adverse effects of inhalation of excessive amounts of nebulized isoproterenol in status asthmaticus. *J. Allergy*, **43**, 101–13
26. Reisman, R. E. (1970). Asthma induced by adrenergic aerosols. *J. Allergy*, **46**, 162–77
27. Sears, M. R. (1991). Dose reduction of beta-agonists in asthma. *Lancet*, **338**, 1331–2

DISCUSSION

Dr D. M. Humphreys (Boehringer Ingelheim, UK) You say that your data relate to regular versus *pro re nata* administration. Surely there is a problem here. Could it not be better expressed as more versus less? After all, '*pro re nata*' used to mean doctors telling their patients to take a drug whenever they felt they needed it. In those circumstances *pro re nata* could become very regular use. If patients are taking two puffs four times a day, this is probably around the maximum recommended dose on the majority of β-agonist data sheets. If people are taking more in addition to that, they are actually exceeding the recommended dose which is supported by the regulatory data submitted for the approval of that licence. There is then the dilemma of whether we are talking about excess dosing or about regular dosing within a recommended range.

Dr M. R. Sears I think it is both. I have not shown the data, but we have patients who have gone from more to less but who are still taking a lot – people who have dropped from 20 puffs a day to ten. They are better on ten puffs, but this is still at least at the upper level of what would be recommended. We have clearly shown that two puffs four times a day is not a good recommendation – this is a recommendation that needs to be re-thought.

Dr N. C. Barnes (London) Your method of analysing the results of the trial is rather unorthodox. If I were setting up a trial comparing essentially treatment A with treatment B, I would compare the peak flow data over the first and second treatment periods. This is the way we understand, and how trials are normally analysed. Has this been done and, if so, what is the result?

Dr M. R. Sears If the morning peak flow data are just analysed as periods A and period B, there is a significant difference in favour of *pro re nata* treatment. All other differences become trends which are no longer significant. However, we chose neither to set up the study nor to analyse the data in that way. The idea of doing a cross-over design was to have patients in both periods of treatment, and look at these markers to get a more sensitive indicator of in which period the control was better. The message is still there, but it is weakened if that analysis is done.

Dr N. C. Barnes What is the magnitude of the difference between the peak flows in the two periods? You said there are non-significant trends. Are those trends all in the direction of regular treatment being worse?

Dr M. R. Sears The mean difference in morning peak flow rates was 10 l/min in favour of higher peak flow rates during as needed treatment.

Dr N. C. Barnes Your analysis has to assign people to either 'better' or 'worse' in one treatment period. There must have been a lot of patients for whom it was more or less even in the two treatment periods or where the differences were so trivial that it would have been difficult to decide. In how many patients was there an absolutely barn-door difference, and in how many was it very difficult to differentiate?

Dr M. R. Sears Seven of the 64 who finished the study could not be allocated. In the other 57, the differences were sufficient to determine a 'better' period. Some of it is random, because asthma fluctuates; if nothing is done, some people will be better in one period than another. In 57 patients, though, the differences were sufficient for them to be allocated to one or other group. Taking a first-pass at the data, looking only at those patients where all the differences point in the same direction, without invoking any hierarchy of importance of markers of control, there is still the same effect. The numbers are smaller, it does not quite achieve the level of significance, but it is there.

7

The Saskatchewan case–control study of β-agonists

W. Spitzer

INTRODUCTION

The Saskatchewan study of β-agonists in asthma is a cohort study which is being analysed, in the first instance, by means of a nested, matched case–control technique.

The importance of acknowledging that this is a cohort study comes from the fact that the cohort logic of observational (or non-experimental) research provides a prospective, forward-looking methodology in which the groups under comparison are delineated by exposure, or by treatment, and are followed forward in time in a way that is analogous to the randomized controlled trial. Indeed, when cohorts are compared, the architecture of the study is as close as it is possible to get to a randomized controlled trial without the study being experimental.

The case–control analysis is nested within the cohort. The strength of the evidence from a cohort is distinctively different from that of a conventional case–control study and the several advantages of this method of analysis will be explained as the data are reviewed.

The study examines the relationship of *any* β-agonist by inhaler with death and near-death; this analysis also compares the two main β-agonists used in Canada, namely, fenoterol and salbutamol.

Part II of the study will consider the clinical implications. In this analysis we will do the best we can in observational research to adjust for the clinical severity of the illness. This part of the analysis is currently nearing completion.

Part III of the study will provide an analysis of the cohort as a cohort. This will enable us to consider absolute rates, attributable rates and rate differences – and these comparisons are, of course, important from the perspective of public health.

It should be noted that Boehringer Ingelheim, who have a distinct commercial interest in one of the products under assessment, sponsored the study. Accordingly, the McGill group required – and this was graciously accepted by the company – that there be a scientific advisory board which would approve the protocol and comment on the results before public submission. The board was chaired by Prof. Ibrahim, Dean of Public Health, University of North Carolina; it included Prof. Kewitz, from Berlin; Prof. Hensley, from Australia; Dr Sheffer, from Harvard University; and Prof. Begaud, from Bordeaux. The statistical and methodological aspects of the peer review were undertaken by Prof. Day, of Cambridge and Prof. Walter, of McMaster University, and additional helpful advice was received from Prof. Burney, of London.

METHODS

The procedures of the study will be described under the following headings: the study population; definition of outcome; definition of the cohort; the asthma drugs under study; concurrent drugs (used as proxies to examine co-morbidity); the nested matched case–control design; the quantification of drug exposure to inhaled fenoterol and salbutamol; other variables for statistical analysis; and the actual statistical analysis.

The study population

The initial screen for potential subjects

The study was carried out in the Canadian province of Saskatchewan. This province is about half the size of Europe and has 1.1 million inhabitants spread from the United States border to the Arctic Circle. There are two cities, each of about 150 000 people, and the rest comprises small towns and farming communities.

A unique feature of Saskatchewan is that all 1.1 million inhabitants are insured for all health services, not by means of a Health Service, as in the UK, but by means of national health insurance. Each individual act of health care is recorded in a computer so that the physicians, hospitals and other providers of care can be paid. The province is further unique, and different from the rest of Canada, in that in addition to the provision of full hospitalization coverage there is also full coverage for payments to physicians and other health care professionals; there is also coverage for the provision of prescription drugs. Each prescription which is dispensed is recorded in the prescription drug plan computer database.

Each resident has a unique identifier for all insurance components of the scheme. This identifier is also valid for the vital statistics files, mortality, births, cancer registry and so on. Linking these databases therefore provides an opportunity to create cohorts, prospective but historically so, with very good evidence of exposure to a drug.

Since prescriptions can be dispensed only every 30 days, there is also a historical record, month by month, of every prescription drug that a patient may have taken. This affords an opportunity for quantification of the exposure to drugs. It is important to note that a patient does not enter the numerator for exposure in the computer database until he has *obtained* the drug. It is not the prescription but the dispensing which provides the exposure measure and this provides much firmer evidence for exposure than a mere record that a prescription has been written.

In identifying the study population, the initial screen for potential subjects involved the review of 20 million prescriptions issued in the period 1980–1987, for persons aged 5–54 years. These prescriptions identified patients who had been dispensed at least one asthma drug, as identified from the prescription drug database and the formularies corresponding to those 8 years. This search yielded 68 813 subjects.

The subset of 'asthmatic' subjects

All of these 68 813 people could not possibly be considered asthmatics. Some patients might have had an isolated prescription for theophylline or even for a β-agonist for some transitory respiratory illness.

A second pass was therefore performed in order to identify those people who had 10 or more dispensed prescriptions for an asthma drug in the same time period (1980–1987). This yielded 12 301 subjects – and these patients became the cohort. We have defined the cohort in this pragmatic way because we were unable to find a universally accepted and useful definition for an asthmatic and, as the study proceeded, the presumption that our cohort was composed of asthmatics was confirmed during the process of validation.

Asthma drugs used to define the population

The drugs used to define the asthmatic population were the following:

(1) Inhaled fenoterol,
(2) Inhaled salbutamol,
(3) Other inhaled β-agonists,
(4) Oral fenoterol,
(5) Oral salbutamol,
(6) Other oral β-agonists,
(7) Theophylline,
(8) Inhaled sodium cromoglycate,
(9) Ipratropium bromide, and
(10) Inhaled corticosteroids.

It should be noted that oral corticosteroids were not used to demarcate the cohort because this would have led to the inclusion of arthritics and other people with chronic diseases who use oral corticosteroids on a long-term basis. Oral corticosteroids were used later in the evaluations, but not to demarcate the population.

Definition of outcomes

The drugs were used to define the cohort. The cohort was therefore defined by exposure, not by outcome, whereas in a conventional case–control study the patient population would be defined by outcome. It is, of course, the outcome which is pursued prospectively in the cohort design or architecture. The scientific advisory board strongly urged the use of asthma-related death plus near-death combined as the primary outcome and, subordinate to that, the subset of asthma-related deaths. Nevertheless, the present data are mainly the mortality data because these are more closely comparable to the earlier work, particularly the studies in New Zealand[1]. Additional data on deaths plus near-deaths will be published shortly.

'Near-death' included severe hypercapnia with or without intubation. The difference between death and near-death can depend solely on factors such as the distance from hospital – and this is why near-death was felt to be part of the same continuum. The sources of data for the identification of outcomes were firstly, the mortality database, comprising death certificates, autopsy reports and coroners' reports. There were 180 deaths in the cohort of 12 301, for which there were records in 165 cases. Some records of deaths are lost because, in Canada, a death out-of-province is imputed to the province of origin. Thus, the fact of a death is known, but often the records themselves are not transmitted. For instance, Quebec will not send to Saskatchewan the records of deaths of people from the latter province who die in Quebec, but will inform Saskatchewan of the death.

Secondly, for the near-deaths, a wide net was cast throughout the entire database of hospitalization with an algorithm designed to yield potential near-deaths by the procedure codes that exist in a fee-for-service insurance system. A total of 1567 patient records were found out of a total of 1581 identified in the computer. After an initial screen we were left with 964 potential subjects.

With regard to the classification of the outcomes, mortality due to all causes was divided into asthma-related mortality and other causes of mortality as being probably, possibly or unlikely to be due to asthma on the basis of an assessment by a panel of experts. This panel comprised three chest physicians from three different universities.

When they unanimously and independently agreed that a death was probably asthma-related, the death was counted as such. It is worth stressing that the drugs used for those patients were removed from all the records employed so that any hidden or overt biases of the chest physicians would be mitigated or eliminated in the process of classification. If there was not a unanimous agreement, a consensus decision was made. In fact, all but four of the cases of death had a unanimous assessment.

Our analysis includes only probable events.

Having taken an analogous approach for the near-deaths, we ended up with 44 asthma-related deaths out of the 165 reviewed and 85 asthma-related near-deaths of the 964 reviewed.

Definition of the cohort

A cohort is easy to understand when all subjects start at the same time; for example, an occupational health study may start with a cohort of 20 000 workers employed in a given year who are then followed forward either concurrently or historically. This is a closed cohort, with approximately the same time zero for all participants. This may also be done with cohorts of patients.

The Saskatchewan study was a dynamic cohort, in which people could enter and exit the cohort at any time during the 8 years. In terms of definition of follow-up, the unit of follow-up is a patient-month of patient-year. The date of the tenth prescription, 1 January 1980 or the date of the fifth birthday was used to define the cohort time of entry. The time of exit was the date of the event, death or the last near-death, emigration, termination, 30 April 1987 or the date of the 55th birthday.

For the 12 301 subjects in the cohort there was also exposure information for the 2 years prior to the inception of the study, so that chronic long-term assessment could be made going back 2 years from the first day covered by the study period.

The asthma drugs under study

The asthma drugs under study, once the cohort had been defined, were the following:

(1) Inhaled fenoterol by metered dose inhaler,
(2) Inhaled salbutamol by metered dose inhaler,
(3) Inhaled fenoterol by nebulizer,
(4) Inhaled salbutamol by nebulizer,
(5) Other inhaled β-agonists,
(6) Oral fenoterol,
(7) Oral salbutamol,
(8) Other oral β-agonists,
(9) Theophylline,
(10) Inhaled sodium cromoglycate,
(11) Ipratropium bromide,
(12) Inhaled corticosteroids, and
(13) Oral corticosteroids.

As part of the prescription drug database there was a month-by-month computer record of all of these drugs, plus any other drug the patients had taken. Several million pieces of data had, therefore, to be examined in undertaking this kind of approach with this size of cohort.

Concurrent drugs used as proxies to examine co-morbidity

There is information in the database on all of the drugs dispensed. The concomitant other (non-asthmatic) drugs were used therefore as proxies for illness (or co-morbidities), that were present in the cohort. The following broad categories, of such drug classes were considered:

(1) Cardiovascular (antihypertensive, potassium-sparing diuretics);

(2) Neurological (anti-convulsants, anti-depressants, tranquillizers);

(3) Contraindicated drugs (β-blockers, sedatives, parasympathomimetics); and

(4) Non-potassium-sparing diuretics.

A composite index of co-morbidity was created by employing all four of these drug classes simultaneously in order to minimize the confounding by severity of illness that might occur in this observational study.

The nested, matched case–control design

A nested case–control analytical design was used. Each of the 129 cases (44 deaths and 85 near-deaths) was individually matched to between two and eight controls; there was a total of 655 controls.

The matching and nesting were undertaken in a way that distinguishes this study from a conventional case–control study; the method used will, therefore, be described in some detail.

The entire cohort of 12 301 asthmatic subjects was divided into two subsets: 129 cases (the 44 deaths and 85 near-deaths) and 12 172 non-cases. The 12 172 non-cases were then divided into 129 subcohorts, each matched to one case. Matching was in terms of the following features:

(1) Region of residence;

(2) Social assistance;

(3) Age at and date of entry into cohort;

(4) Presence of a hospitalization in 2 years prior to index date; and

(5) Controls must have been at risk at same time as their matched case (i.e. at index date).

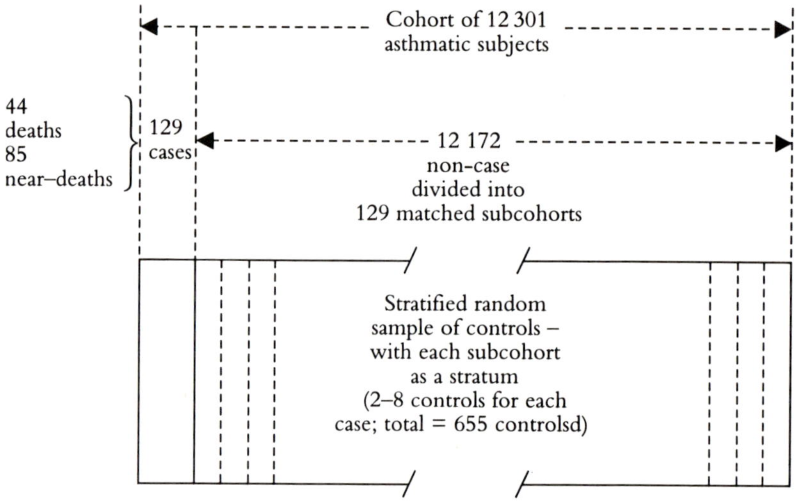

Figure 1 Method of nesting the probability sample within the cohort used in this study

From each of these 129 subcohorts a probability sample of up to eight controls per case was drawn (sometimes there were only two in the subcohorts that could be matched to an individual case). The controls (total 655) were therefore a probability sample of the non-cases that rendered the analysis theoretically identical – and this has been proved empirically – to analysing the study as a cohort. Instead of having to analyse 12 172 controls only 655 have had to be analysed, in keeping with the conventional approaches of sampling. Thus, this method of analysis has been highly efficient. Figure 1 shows how the probability sample was nested within the cohort.

It will be seen that there was a total of 784 case–control study subjects (129 cases and 655 controls).

The quantification of exposure to inhaled fenoterol and salbutamol by metered dose inhaler

Due to the characteristics of the prescription drug database it was possible to establish three different measures of drug use; that is of exposure to fenoterol and salbutamol administered by metered dose inhaler.

One measure was dichotomous: it was possible to measure the presence or absence of exposure in the last 12 months. It is worth stressing that this study is focused on chronic, not acute, exposure – exposure over the entire prior 12 months, not the recent experience immediately prior to the outcome event.

The second was an ordinal measure giving graded levels of exposure. This analysis permitted as assessment of dose response. This is clearly important in trying to determine the causal significance of the findings. Exposure was graded into:

(1) The use of zero units (on metered dose inhaler) per year (a reference standard that would give an odds ratio of 1);

(2) 1–12 units per year (an average of 0–1 canisters per month), representing moderately low use;

(3) 13–24 units per year (an average of 1–2 canisters per month), representing moderately high use but still within the dose limits allowed by the prescribing information.

(4) Over 24 units per year – an excessively high use.

The third strategy of analysis provided a continuous measure of exposure and looked at linear dose–response relationships. Among the deaths no subject failed to receive a β-agonist. The continuous measure of exposure considered the actual number of units used per month. Thus, the relevant odds ratios are per unit of use. For example, the odds ratios 1 unit versus 0 units per month, 2 units versus 1 per month – and so on. In this context, 1 unit equals 1 metered dose inhaler per month or its equivalent.

Other variables for statistical analysis

Other variables were used for statistical analysis in order to render the groups being compared as similar as possible, given that we were conducting an observational study. The co-factors available in the Saskatchewan databases with which to standardize the calculated odds ratios included:

(1) The use of other drugs (it is important, for instance, when considering just fenoterol and salbutamol (and ignoring for the moment, terbutaline and the other drugs examined) to see what happens to patients who use say, fenoterol with salbutamol given either concomitantly, before or

after the fenoterol; it is also necessary to consider the number of prescriptions for theophylline, the presence or absence of an oral or inhaled corticosteroid, and the use of sodium cromoglycate);

(2) The number of physician and specialist visits in the last 24 months;

(3) The number of hospitalizations in the last 24 months;

(4) The number of co-therapy categories; and

(5) The index of co-morbidity (which has been described earlier).

The actual statistical analysis

The main analyses involved conditional logistic multiple regression. The models used were carefully verified for validity and robustness. Their stability was also looked at by including and excluding extreme values at either end, and assessing what difference this made to the findings.

RESULTS

The number of hospitalizations for asthma in the 2 years prior to the index date

The findings (Table 1) demonstrate the importance of undertaking the kind of adjustments that have been mentioned. The number of hospitalizations for asthma in the last 2 years prior to the index date (whether deaths alone

Table 1 The number of hospitalizations for asthma in the 2 years prior to the index date

	Deaths and near-deaths		*Deaths*	
	Cases	*Controls*	*Cases*	*Controls*
n	129	655	44	233
No. of hospitalizations for asthma				
mean	2.1	1.0	2.5	1.2
median	1.0	1.0	1.0	1.0
range	0–21	0–8	0–15	0–8
standard deviation	3.4	1.3	3.6	1.4

Table 2 Use of health services in the 2 years prior to the index date

	Deaths and near-deaths		*Deaths*	
	Cases	*Controls*	*Cases*	*Controls*
n	129	655	44	233
No. of specialist visits*				
mean	9.7	5.9	7.1	5.3
median	5.0	1.0	3.0	2.0
range	0–62	0–80	0–62	0–80
standard deviation	11.2	9.7	10.9	10.2
No. of non-specialist visits				
mean	34.7	25.5	39.3	26.5
median	27.0	18.0	30.0	19.0
range	2–204	0–173	4–204	0–110
standard deviation	30.0	24.4	37.4	24.5

*Specialists in respirology, allergy, paediatrics and internal medicine

or deaths plus near-deaths were investigated) was a little more than twice as high among the cases than the controls. This means that there has to be an adjustment for hospitalization in looking at the final odds ratios.

The use of health services in the 2 years prior to the index date

Likewise, the use of specialists in respiratory medicine, allergy, paediatrics and internal medicine, was higher among cases than controls (Table 2). Similarly, the use was appreciably higher for general family physicians among cases than controls. This again, shows that there has to be adjustment for this variable in determining the final results of the study.

Concomitant use of drugs (co-therapy) during the 12 months prior to the index date

In respect of deaths alone (Table 3), there was a trend, both for cardiovascular and for neurological drugs, which resulted in a non-significantly higher odds ratio. For contraindicated drugs, there was a statistically significant effect, as there was for the overall index of co-morbidity – again showing that adjustment had to be made for the use of other drugs in presenting the final odds ratios on the β-agonists.

Table 3 Use of drugs in co-therapy during the 12 months prior to the index date

	Deaths					
	Cases		*Controls*			
Drug exposure	*Yes*	*No*	*Yes*	*No*	*OR**	*95% CI†*
Cardiovascular	7	37	19	214	2.2	0.8–5.8
Neurological	5	39	14	219	2.2	0.7–7.2
Contraindicated	10	34	27	206	2.5	1.0–6.2
Diuretic	8	36	23	210	2.2	0.9–5.4
Index of co-morbidity	15	29	48	185	2.2	1.0–4.9

*OR, odds ratio; †95% confidence intervals

Table 4 Distribution of fenoterol and salbutamol dose exposure by metered dose inhaler in the 12 months prior to the index date

	Fenoterol		*Salbutamol*	
	Cases	*Controls*	*Cases*	*Controls*
Deaths and near-deaths				
n	42	83	99	444
mean	26.6	16.0	20.1	13.1
range	1–106	1–67	1–82	1–70
standard deviation	21.1	14.7	17.8	12.0
Deaths				
n	21	37	28	156
mean	34.1	13.2	16.3	12.1
range	4–106	1–56	1–50	1–50
standard deviation	23.7	11.9	14.8	11.5

Distribution of fenoterol and salbutamol dose exposure by metered dose inhaler in the prior 12 months

An interesting finding, that reflects the varying patterns of practice in Saskatchewan, was that there were cases with remarkably high usage of specific antiasthma drugs (Table 4). For example, one patient received 106 canisters of fenoterol in a year. For salbutamol, the upper limit of the range was 82 canisters per year for deaths plus near-deaths and 50 canisters per year among patients who died. This shows very high use among some of these subjects. Even among controls (that is asthmatics who did not die) there were some patients using between 50 and 70 metered dose inhalers over the 12-month period.

Simple matched odds ratio of adverse event for presence or absence of exposure to asthma drugs during the 12-month period prior to the index date

Table 5 is perhaps most similar to the key table in the first of the Wellington studies[3]. First, it should be noted that there were no deaths who failed to have a β-agonist. This zero cell in respect of the measure 'any β-agonist' is the continuous model was used to assess this parameter.

Table 5 presents what are unadjusted, nearly raw, data. The fact that they are matched means that the data are not quite raw but they are nearly so.

Table 5 Simple matched odds ratio (OR) of adverse event for presence or absence of asthma drug exposure during the 12 months prior to the index date; 95% confidence intervals (CI) are also shown

	Deaths					
	Cases		*Controls*			
Exposure	*Yes*	*No*	*Yes*	*No*	*OR*	*95% CI*
Any inhaled β-agonist	44	0	192	41	NE*	NE
fenoterol	21	23	37	196	5.3	2.5–11.5
by metered dose inhaler	21	23	37	196	5.3	2.5–11.5
by nebulizer†	0	44	1	232	NE	NE
salbutamol	30	14	160	73	1.0	0.5–2.0
by metered dose inhaler	28	16	156	77	0.9	0.5–1.7
by nebulizer	7	37	15	217	3.5	1.1–10.9
other†	1	43	16	218	0.4	0.05–2.7
Any oral β-agonist	20	24	74	159	1.8	0.9–3.5
Theophylline	35	9	125	108	3.7	1.6–8.4
Inhaled corticosteroids	22	22	81	152	1.8	0.9–3.6
Oral corticosteroids	24	20	72	161	3.1	1.5–6.5
Cromolyn	17	27	67	166	1.6	0.8–3.3

*NE, not estimable; †frequencies too low for all further analyses presented in this report

Table 6 Adjusted matched odds ratios (OR) and 95% confidence intervals (CI) for presence versus absence of exposure during 12 months for inhaled β-agonists

	Deaths and near-deaths		*Deaths*	
Exposure	*OR*	*95% CI*	*OR*	*95% CI*
Fenoterol by metered dose inhaler	6.1	3.1–12.2	9.1	3.0–28.1
Salbutamol by metered dose inhaler	4.1	2.1–8.0	2.8	1.0–7.6
Salbutamol by nebulizer	2.5	1.2–5.5	3.0	0.7–13.1
Other inhaled β-agonist	2.6	1.1–6.2	NE*	NE

*NE, not estimable

There are no adjustments, either for one another or for all the factors for which it has been noted that adjustment should be made.

In the patients who died there was an odds ratio of 5.3 for fenoterol (compared to 1.55 in the first Wellington case–control study), and 0.9 for salbutamol by metered dose inhaler (compared to 0.7 found in Wellington). However, these findings, like theirs, are not adjusted for the other drugs taken. The Wellington group's standardization was by stratification, which is a very different approach to that of regression. The raw finding of an odds ratio of 3.7 for theophylline in this study is of interest.

Adjusted matched odds ratios for presence versus absence of exposure to β-agonists during 12 months

When these raw findings in respect of asthma deaths were adjusted for all the influential co-variables that have been mentioned, the odds ratios for fenoterol and salbutamol given by metered dose inhalers went up to 9.1 (95% confidence intervals 3.0–28.1) and 2.8 (95% confidence intervals 1.0–7.6) respectively (Table 6). The odds ratios were also fairly high when both the deaths and near-deaths were considered. When the adjustments were made the odds ratio in the fatal cases for theophylline stayed around 3, and the confidence intervals included unity (Table 7).

These same adjusted matched odds ratios for the presence or absence of exposure to theophylline were 3.3 in the deaths and 2.4 in the deaths plus near-deaths with, in both instances, the confidence intervals excluding unity. These odds ratios for the β-agonists are in the range in which they would impress most epidemiologists.

Table 7 Adjusted matched odds ratios (OR) and 95% confidence intervals (CI) for presence versus absence of exposure during 12 months for other treatments

	Deaths and near-deaths		*Deaths*	
Exposure	*OR*	*95% CI*	*OR*	*95% CI*
Any oral β-agonist	1.5	0.9–2.5	2.3	0.9–5.6
Theophylline	2.4	1.4–4.3	3.3	1.3–8.8
Oral corticosteroids	2.6	1.5–4.4	1.2	0.5–2.9
Inhaled corticosteroids or cromolyn	1.3	0.8–2.1	1.6	0.7–3.5

Table 8 Adjusted matched odds ratios (OR) and 95% confidence intervals (CI) for ordinal classification of exposure

	Deaths	
Units dispensed	*OR*	*95% CI*
Fenoterol by metered dose inhaler		
0	1.0	
1–12	4.7	1.1–20.6
13–24	40.5	5.1–319
25 +	113.2	17.0–754
Salbutamol by metered dose inhaler		
0	1.0	
1–12	3.4	0.9–13.3
13–24	10.0	2.1–46.5
25 +	29.4	5.1–171

Adjusted matched odds ratios for the ordinal classification of exposure

The odds ratios given in Table 8 for the ordinal classification of exposure were adjusted for one another and for all of the other factors previously enumerated. Fenoterol had an odds ratio of 4.7 and salbutamol 3.4 when these agents were given within the therapeutic range by metered dose inhalers. The odds ratios for higher doses of fenoterol and salbutamol were 40 and 10, respectively. When 25 or more canisters were used per year then the odds ratios were 113 and 30 for fenoterol and salbutamol, respectively. All of these odds ratios had lower confidence intervals which exceeded unity.

Table 9 Adjusted matched odds ratios (OR) and 95% confidence intervals (CI) for ordinal classification of exposure during the 12 months prior to the index date

	Deaths	
	OR	*95% CI*
Fenoterol by metered dose inhaler		
0	1.0	
1–6	3.1	0.5–20.4
7–12	9.0	1.1–73.1
13 +	90.0	15.2–533
Salbutamol by metered dose inhaler		
0	1.0	
1–12	4.4	1.1–17.1
13–24	13.1	2.7–64.3
25 +	40.3	6.2–260

Adjusted matched odds ratios for the ordinal classification of exposure during the prior 12 months

Fenoterol has been marketed in Canada in a metered dose inhaler delivering 200 μg per activation; the salbutamol inhaler delivers 100 μg, and these dosage forms were in use during the entire time span covered by this study. The data are corrected for the number of canisters that would deliver the same amount of the active principle in Table 9.

In this table, 1–6 units has been adjusted to be equivalent to 1–12, and 7–12 to be equivalent to 13–24 units. Again, the odds, ratio ranged from 1 to 3, 9 and 90, for fenoterol and 1 to 4, 13 and 40 for salbutamol, respectively, as the number of units used per year increased. The confidence intervals around these odds ratios were wide but at the highest of the two dose levels considered, they excluded unity.

Adjusted matched odds ratios for treatment during the prior 12 months

The third strategy of analysis regarding drug exposure was the continuous or dose–response approach – and this determines the amount by which the risk rises per additional canister taken per month. For fenoterol the relevant odds ratio was 5.4 – clearly statistically significant – and for salbutamol it

Table 10 Adjusted matched odds ratios (OR) and 95% confidence intervals (CI) for treatment during the 12 months prior to the index date

	Deaths	
Exposure	*OR*	*95% CI*
Fenoterol by metered dose inhaler (units per month)	5.4	2.4–11.8
Salbutamol by metered dose inhaler (units per month)	2.4	1.5–3.8
Fenoterol by metered dose inhaler (per 100 μg)	2.3	1.6–3.4

was 2.4, which was also statistically significant. When a microgram per microgram adjustment was made the odds ratio per 100 μg, for fenoterol by metered dose inhaler, became 2.3 (95% confidence interval 1.6–3.4) (Table 10).

Adjusted matched odds ratios per unit per month of exposure during the 12 months prior to the index date

Relating to the primary hypothesis: any inhaled β-agonist; because of the cells containing zero in the earlier analysis, the only way to look at this problem was by means of the continuous model. For deaths plus near-deaths, the odds ratio was doubled when metered dose inhalers per month were considered for any β-agonist; for deaths alone the odds ratio was 2.6 (95% confidence interval 1.7–3.9), while for deaths plus near-deaths the odds ratio was 2.0 (95% confidence interval 1.6–2.4).

Adjusted matched odds ratios for exposure (treatment) during the 12-month period prior to the index date or event

For inhaled beclomethasone, the odds ratio was 0.1 for taking 12 or more canisters per month; in order words, for regular use. This suggests a very highly protective and clearly statistically significant effect of oral corticosteroids. Cromolyn had a trend in the same direction but there were insufficient numbers fully to establish this finding. When these results were combined (as in Table 11), the trend was even clearer and odds ratios of 1.5 and 0.6 for using 1–5 or ≥ 6 units, respectively were found. However, it

Table 11 Adjusted matched odds ratios (OR) and 95% confidence intervals (CI) for treatment during the 12 months prior to the index date

	Deaths and near-deaths	
Exposure	*OR*	*95% CI*
Fenoterol by metered dose inhaler (units per month)	2.3	1.7–3.1
Salbutamol by metered dose inhaler (units per month)	1.9	1.5–2.4
Inhaled corticosteroids or cromolyn units over 12 months		
0	1.0	
1–5	1.5	0.8–2.6
6 +	0.6	0.3–1.2
Fenoterol by metered dose inhaler (per 100 μg)	1.5	1.3–1.8

should be noted that the confidence intervals around both of these ratios included unity.

This is probably as important a result as any in our study. The additional importance of this finding is that if every drug studied had showed odds ratios increasing in the same direction then it would very strongly suggest that all we were looking at was confounding by severity. The fact that at least this one class of drug has odds ratios moving in the opposite direction does not exclude this possibility, but it militates against it.

DISCUSSION

One might seek explanations for increased risk of adverse events apparently associated with the use of β-agonists.

β-agonists may be a cause of the problem, or they may be a marker of severity of the illness. In observational studies it is not possible to be quite sure which of these two explanations is the true one. Certainly this cannot be sorted out totally in this study, and it may not be possible to do so even after Parts II and III of the analysis are completed and when the clinical results are available.

What may be called the 'life-jacket' problem may be happening. If a case–control study of drowning were done and life-jackets used as an exposure assessment, there would probably be a high odds ratio for life-jackets – because they are thrown at people who are drowning. This is perhaps similar to what is happening here.

We think that this is not likely to be the entire explanation, however. Looking at the information excluding the last 4 months prior to the fatal or near-fatal event, taking only chronic exposure distal from the event by at least 4 months (from month 12 to month 8) into account, the odds ratios were similar, somewhat lower, but still statistically significant.

Taking the non-hospitalized subset in the cohort, and excluding anybody who had had a hospitalization – in order to get a lower risk type of cohort – again showed that the odds ratios, whilst lower, remained mostly statistically significant and are clinically important.

Both of the factors now being considered may be operative, and β-agonists may act partly as a marker for severity of disease, and partly a causative factor in asthma deaths and near-deaths.

To the clinician it does not really matter whether these increased and dose-related odds ratios are a marker for severity of disease or an indicator that the drug causes an increased number of deaths or near-deaths – or that both factors are operating. What matters is that a patient who is taking more than two canisters a month is at a marked increased risk of death or near-death and that this is not the situation with inhaled corticosteroids or cromoglycate.

My own personal view is that the elucidation of cause or marker effect will require a mosaic of further studies, including controlled trials and mechanistic studies. While these studies are put into effect, clinicians, regulators and pharmaceutical companies should, I believe, note that when an asthmatic is taking an average of more than 1 or 2 canisters per month of β-agonists, then that patient should be under very careful surveillance.

CONCLUSIONS

The interim conclusions are as follows:

(1) The use of inhaled β-agonists by metered dose inhaler is associated with excess asthma deaths and near-deaths. The distinctive finding of this study, in contrast to the important Wellington studies which signalled this problem to the world[1], is that we think that a class action is being observed, as opposed to the action of one particular drug.

(2) It is important to note that a gradient of risk is observed for both fenoterol and salbutamol. This strongly suggests that we are looking at a true drug-related effect in which it would be expected that a dose–response phenomenon would be observed. For exposures in excess of the recommended dose the risks are notably high – more so for fenoterol than for salbutamol.

(3) On a weight equivalent basis (μg/μg) the risks appear similar for both drugs within the therapeutic range, but are worse for fenoterol outside the therapeutic range.

(4) The risks of most drugs used in the treatment of asthma seem appreciably elevated.

(5) Inhaled topical anti-inflammatory agents (inhaled corticosteroids and cromoglycates) exhibit a trend which, when the results for both kinds of drugs are considered together suggests a protective effect. This finding militates against the possibility that the results of this study are due simply to confounding by the severity of the asthma in patients being treated with these medications.

ACKNOWLEDGEMENTS

My co-workers in this study have included Samy Suissa, Pierre Ernst, Ralph Horwitz, Brian Habbick, Donald Cockcroft, Jean-Francois Boivin, Mary McNutt, A. Sonia Buist and Anthony Rebuck and it is a pleasure to record my gratitude to all those who have contributed to the design and execution of this exercise. Dr Ronald Mann edited the initial longer transcript of this address for the Royal Society of Medicine.

REFERENCE

1. Crane, J., Pearce, N. E., Flatt, A. *et al.* (1989). Prescribed fenoterol and death from asthma in New Zealand, 1981–1983: case–control study. *Lancet*, **1**, 917–22

DISCUSSION

Dr R. Fuller (Glaxo) Obviously, your odds ratios are very high and ostensibly very worrying, but there were only 44 deaths in 8 years in 1 million patients. What are the overall deaths both for asthma and associated with the drugs in the study to put this into context?

Dr W. Spitzer The absolute rates are low. We are still in the process of adjusting them. The important finding here in terms of absolute rates is the attributable risk for excess use in overall-use of β-agonist and so on. The analysis is not quite finished, and I can give only raw data.

Dr P. Howarth (UK) Would you comment further on the nebulizer data? Obviously the dose of β-agonist given by nebulizer is considerably greater than that given by a metered dose inhaler, yet the odds ratios did not look as worrying as with the excessive metered dose inhaler use.

Dr W. Spitzer That is an interesting observation. I could not comment on all the conundrums that have arisen. There may be a component in the ultimate effects observed that is mediated either by unsupervised use of drugs or their improper use as recommended by certain general practitioners or physicians. It would seem that when nebulized drugs are used in Saskatchewan, the supervision – by qualified specialists and so on – is such that this intervening factor may be playing a part. This is speculation; the numbers came out the way they did, and this is the only explanation we could think of drawing from these computerized data.

This gives me the excuse to indicate that in no circumstances do we wish to throw out the baby with the bath-water. These bronchodilators are extremely important rescue medications; they are essential in the armamentarium for physicians in casualty rooms, and seem to be much less of a problem when used in that context.

At the end of the discussion it was stated that Dr Spitzer's paper will appear in the *New England Journal of Medicine*, 20 February 1992.

8

Different patterns of asthma mortality and their association with β-agonist therapy

R. Beasley, N. Pearce, C. Burgess and J. Crane

INTRODUCTION

To understand the relationship between β-agonist drugs and asthma mortality, it is necessary to examine the history of the association, and not just focus on current issues. In particular, two different patterns of asthma mortality have occurred internationally during the last 30 years. There were epidemics of asthma mortality in six countries in the 1960s, and a second epidemic in New Zealand in the late 1970s. Separate from these epidemics, there has also been a more gradual background increase in asthma mortality during the last 20 years, a trend which has been observed in many countries, irrespective of whether they have also experienced an asthma mortality epidemic. Thus, two distinct patterns of increased asthma mortality have been observed, and to understand better their possible relationship with β-agonist drug therapy, they need to be considered separately.

THE FIRST ASTHMA MORTALITY EPIDEMIC

In the 1960s, sudden epidemics of asthma deaths occurred in six countries including Australia, New Zealand, England and Wales[1]. The epidemics did not occur in other countries such as the United States and West Germany, and were unexpected, since death rates had been relatively stable since the turn of the century[2]. Initially, attention focused on the use of β-agonist aerosols in general, the sales of which had increased markedly following their introduction in the early 1960s[3]. However, there were some major anomalies in this general hypothesis, particularly as sales of β-agonist aerosols were very high in the United States, a country in which there had been no epidemic. The situation was clarified by Stolley who noted that a high-dose preparation of isoprenaline (isoprenaline forte) which contained five times the dose per actuation of other isoprenaline preparations, had only been marketed in eight countries. Six of these had mortality epidemics which coincided with the introduction of the drug and in the other two countries (the Netherlands and Belgium) this preparation was introduced relatively late and sales volumes were low[1]. No epidemics occurred in countries where isoprenaline forte was not marketed. There was a strong positive correlation between the asthma mortality rates and isoprenaline forte sales in the eight countries in which isoprenaline forte was available[4].

As a result of this and other evidence, isoprenaline forte was generally considered to be the cause of the asthma mortality epidemic. Death from bronchodilator aerosols was designated one of the most important adverse drug reactions since thalidomide[5], and a British Medical Journal editorial entitled 'Asthma deaths: a question answered' concluded that '[Stolley's work] strengthens still further the case for relating the increase in asthma deaths to aerosols and the sympathomimetic drugs they contain'[6]. The mortality rate declined following warnings from regulatory bodies in different countries, a marked reduction in the sales of isoprenaline forte, and other changes in medical practice, such as an increase in hospital admissions and increasing use of oral corticosteroids.

THE SECOND ASTHMA MORTALITY EPIDEMIC

In 1976 a second asthma mortality epidemic occurred in New Zealand but not in other countries. A national asthma mortality survey was undertaken, but no clear explanation for the epidemic was identified, and conflicting statements were made with respect to the possible role of β-agonist therapy. The initial report[7] stated that 'excessive use of bronchodilator drugs did not account for the high mortality rates' whereas a later report[8] from the same study stated that 'excessive reliance on bronchodilator therapy was the most likely explanation for the epidemic'. Perhaps the strongest evidence against a causal association with β-agonist use in general, was that the steep increase in total sales of inhaled β-agonist drugs in New Zealand commenced in 1980, 4 years after the asthma mortality epidemic had begun[9].

In contrast to the relationship with total β-agonist sales, there was a close association between the introduction and increasing sales of the β-agonist fenoterol and the increase in asthma deaths in New Zealand[10]. Fenoterol, which was marketed as a high-dose preparation and which has similar properties to isoprenaline[11], was introduced in 1976, the year the epidemic started, and mortality tripled in the following 4 years, during which it achieved a stable 30% market share[10]. In contrast, fenoterol represented less than 5% of the market share in most other countries, and in those countries such as West Germany in which it had a high market share, the *per capita* sales were considerably less than those in New Zealand.

Following this and other epidemiological[12] and experimental[13] evidence, the possible role of fenoterol in the New Zealand asthma mortality epidemic was investigated by undertaking a series of three case–control studies[10,14,15]. In each of these studies, which employed different methods and incorporated different data sources, at different time periods throughout the epidemic, an increased risk of asthma death was found in asthmatic patients prescribed fenoterol. The association between fenoterol and asthma deaths was particularly strong in subgroups with more severe asthma, a pattern which essentially rules out the possibility that the findings are due to confounding by severity[16]. In other words, this pattern indicates that the findings were not due to any tendency for more severe patients to be preferentially prescribed fenoterol.

More recently a similar case–control study from Saskatchewan, undertaken specifically to address the 'fenoterol hypothesis' has also found that the prescription of fenoterol was associated with an increased risk of death compared with the more commonly prescribed β-agonist salbutamol[17]. Although the authors also raised the possibility of a general β-agonist class effect, their inability to control for asthma severity when investigating a possible class effect, means that these findings should be regarded as preliminary. To investigate the possibility of a general β-agonist class effect, a case–control study of asthma mortality and prescription of salbutamol at the time of its introduction and increasing use in New Zealand (1969–1975) was recently undertaken, using the same methods as employed in the fenoterol studies[18]. In this very small study, little evidence of an increased risk was found with salbutamol, which is consistent with the observations that mortality fell at the time of its introduction into New Zealand.

By their nature, epidemiological studies such as those discussed are unable to identify the underlying mechanisms by which the high-dose preparations of isoprenaline and fenoterol led to the increased risk of death. Although the mechanism(s) will need to be further investigated in experimental studies, there is already considerable evidence that isoprenaline and fenoterol lead to greater adverse cardiovascular effects than other commonly used β-agonist drugs when inhaled repeatedly by asthmatic subjects[19,20], and that these effects may be particularly harmful in the clinical situation of hypoxia[21].

GRADUAL INCREASE IN ASTHMA MORTALITY

A separate feature of the international trends in asthma mortality has been the gradual increase that has occurred in many countries during the last 20 years[22]. This background increase has occurred not only in countries which have experienced the sudden epidemics, but also in those which did not have high sales of isoprenaline or fenoterol, and have consistently had low mortality rates.

Investigation of the possible relationship between β-agonist therapy and this gradual trend of increasing asthma mortality over such a long period of time is inherently difficult due to the many non-pharmacological factors, which may have led to more severe asthma within the community[23,24]. There are also many aspects of medical practice not directly related to β-agonist therapy which have changed over this long period, and which make the interpretation of changes in asthma mortality difficult.

Despite these problems of interpretation it should be noted that in several countries a close correlation has been observed between increasing mortality and morbidity from asthma and sales of β-agonist drugs[24–26]. It is not clear, however, whether this relationship is due to the increasing use of β-agonist drugs leading to increased bronchial hyper-responsiveness, as has been shown with a number of β-agonist drugs[27–29], or to more severe clinical asthma, thus far suggested solely with adrenaline[30], isoprenaline[31] and fenoterol[27]. Alternative possibilities are that the increase in the use of β-agonist drugs has been in response to an increase in the prevalence of severe asthma due to unrelated non-pharmacological factors, or has been merely the result of aggressive marketing by pharmaceutical companies.

Clearly further studies will be required to clarify these hypotheses, although it will be very difficult to address these issues in epidemiological studies, because the widespread use of β-agonists makes it difficult to identify an appropriate comparison group. Randomized clinical trials will be necessary to address these hypotheses adequately, and to determine whether the possible problems associated with long-term β-agonist therapy may also apply to other bronchodilator drugs[32].

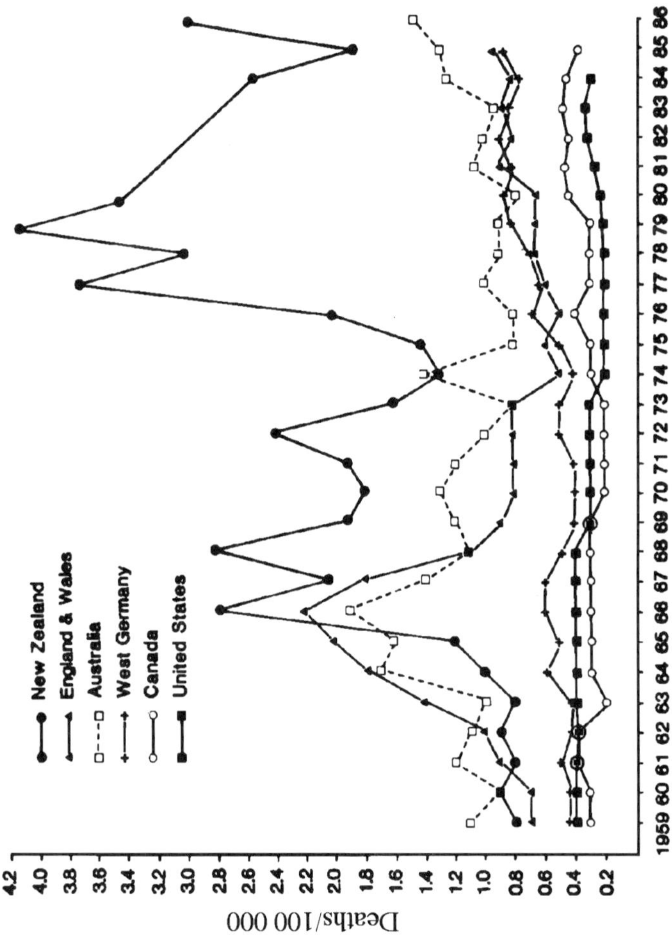

Figure 1 Asthma mortality (per 100 000) in 5–34 year olds in a number of different countries during the last 30 years, showing the different trends. (Reproduced from reference 33 with permission)

CONCLUSION

The epidemics of asthma mortality that occurred in a number of countries in the 1960s and in New Zealand in the 1970s are most likely to have been due to the use of the high-dose preparations of the potent β-agonist drugs isoprenaline and fenoterol respectively. In both epidemics, the mortality rate subsequently fell after warnings about the safety of these agents, restrictions of their use by regulatory authorities, and other changes in management. No other β-agonist drugs have been incriminated in asthma mortality epidemics. In contrast, the cause of the more gradual increase in asthma mortality that has been observed in many countries over recent decades is not clear. One of the many possibilities is that it relates to the increasing use of β-agonist drugs.

What is now evident is that the role of β-agonist therapy requires urgent reappraisal, both in the management of the individual with reversible airways obstruction and in the broader public health context. Such reappraisal needs to consider differences between individual drugs as well as class effects, and should be based on careful clinical and epidemiological studies.

REFERENCES

1. Stolley, P. D. (1972). Asthma mortality: why the United States was spared an epidemic of deaths due to asthma. *Am. Rev. Respir. Dis.*, **105**, 883–90
2. Speizer, F. E. and Doll, R. (1968). A century of asthma deaths in young people. *Br. Med. J.*, **3**, 245–6
3. Inman, W. H. W. and Adelstein, A. M. (1969). Rise and fall of asthma mortality in England and Wales in relation to use of pressurised aerosols. *Lancet*, **2**, 279–85
4. Stolley, P. D. and Schinnar, R. (1978). Association between asthma mortality and isoproterenol: a review. *Prev. Med.*, **7**, 519–38
5. Venning, G. R. (1983). Identification of adverse reactions to new drugs. I. What have been the important adverse reactions since thalidomide? *Br. Med. J.*, **286**, 199–202
6. Editorial. (1972). Asthma deaths. A question answered. *Br. Med. J.*, **2**, 443–4
7. Sears, M. R., Rea, H. H., Beaglehole, R., Gillies, A. J. D., Holst, P. E., O'Donnell, T. V., Rothwell, R. P. G. and Sutherland, D. C. (1985). Asthma mortality in New Zealand: a two year national study. *N. Z. Med. J.*, **98**, 271–5

8. Beaglehole, R., Jackson, R., Sears, M. and Rea, H. (1987). Asthma mortality in New Zealand: a review with some policy implications. *N. Z. Med. J.*, **100**, 231–4
9. Keating, G., Mitchell, E. A., Jackson, R., Beaglehole, R. and Rea, H. (1984). Trends in sales of drugs for asthma in New Zealand, Australia and the United Kingdom, 1975–81. *Br. Med. J.*, **289**, 348–51
10. Crane, J., Pearce, N., Flatt, A., Burgess, C., Jackson, R., Kwong, T., Ball, M. and Beasley, R. (1989). Prescribed fenoterol and death from asthma in New Zealand, 1981–83: case–control study. *Lancet*, **1**, 917–22
11. Crane, J., Burgess, C. and Beasley, R. (1989). Cardiovascular and hypokalaemic effects of inhaled salbutamol, fenoterol and isoprenaline. *Thorax*, **44**, 136–40
12. Pearce, N., Crane, J., Burgess, C., Jackson, R. and Beasley, R. (1991). Beta agonists and asthma mortality: déjà vu. *Clin. Exp. Allergy*, **21**, 401–10
13. Beasley, R., Pearce, N., Crane, J., Windon, H. and Burgess, C. (1991). Asthma mortality and inhaled beta agonist therapy. *Aust. N. Z. J. Med.*, **21**, 753–63
14. Pearce, N., Grainger, J., Atkinson, M., Crane, J., Burgess, C., Culling, C., Windom, H. and Beasley, R. (1990). Case–control study of prescribed fenoterol and death from asthma in New Zealand, 1977–1981. *Thorax*, **45**, 170–5
15. Grainger, J., Woodman, K., Pearce, N., Crane, J., Burgess, C., Keane, A. and Beasley, R. (1991). Prescribed fenoterol and death from asthma in New Zealand, 1981–1987: a further case control study. *Thorax*, **46**, 105–11
16. Sackett, D. L., Shannon, H. S. and Browman, G. W. (1990). Fenoterol and fatal asthma. *Lancet*, **1**, 45–6
17. Spitzer, W. D., Suissa, S., Ernst, P., Horwitz, R. I., Habbick, B., Cockcroft, D., Bovin, J. F., McNutt, M., Buist, A. S. and Rebuck, A. (1992). The use of beta agonists and the risk of death and near death from asthma. *N. Engl. J. Med.*, **326**, 501–6
18. Woodman, K., Beasley, R., Pearce, N., Burgess, C. and Crane, J. (1992). Salbutamol and asthma deaths in New Zealand, 1969–1970. Case–control study. *Clin. Pharmacol. Ther.*, in press
19. Wong, C. S., Pavord,. I. D., Williams, J., Britton, J. R. and Tattersfield, A. E. (1990). Bronchodilator, cardiovascular and hypokalaemic effects of fenoterol, salbutamol and terbutaline in asthma. *Lancet*, **336**, 1396–9
20. Windom, H., Burgess, C., Siebers, R., Crane, J., Purdie, G. and Beasley, R. (1990). The pulmonary and extrapulmonary effects of inhaled beta agonists in asthmatic patients. *Clin. Pharmacol. Ther.*, **48**, 296–301

21. Collins, J. M., McDevitt, D. G., Shanks, R. G. and Swanton, J. G. (1969). The cardiotoxicity of isoprenaline during hypoxia. *Br. J. Pharmacol.*, **36**, 35–45
22. Jackson, R., Sears, M. R., Beaglehole, R. and Rea, H. H. (1988). International trends in asthma mortality: 1970 to 1985. *Chest*, **94**, 914–18
23. Commentary (1990). Asthma. *J. Epidemiol. Commun. Health*, **44**, 177–8
24. Mitchell, E. (1989). Is current treatment increasing asthma mortality and morbidity. *Thorax*, **44**, 81–4
25. Hay, I. F. C. and Higenbottam, T. (1987). Has the management of asthma improved? *Lancet*, **2**, 609–11
26. Jenkins, M. A., Hurley, S. F., Bowes, G. and McNeil, J. J. (1990). Use of anti-asthmatic drugs in Australia. *Med. J. Aust.*, **153**, 323–8
27. Sears, M. R., Taylor, D. R., Print, C. G., Lake, D. C., Quigqing, L., Flannery, E. M., Yates, D. M., Lucas, M. K. and Herbison, G. P. (1990). Regular inhaled beta-agonist treatment in bronchial asthma. *Lancet*, **336**, 1391–6
28. Vathenen, A. S., Knox, A. J., Higgins, B. G., Britton, J. R. and Tattersfield, A. E. (1988). Rebound increase in bronchial responsiveness after treatment with inhaled terbutaline. *Lancet*, **1**, 554–8
29. van Schayck, C. P., Graafsma, S. J., Visch, M. B., Dompeling, E., van Weel, C. and van Herwaarden, C. L. A. (1990). Increased bronchial hyperresponsiveness after inhaling salbutamol during 1 year is not caused by sensitisation to salbutamol. *J. Allergy Clin. Immunol.*, **86**, 793–800
30. Benson, R. L. and Perlman, F. (1948). Clinical effects of epinephrine by inhalation. *J. Allergy*, **19**, 129–40
31. van Metre, T. E. (1969). Adverse effects of inhalation of excessive amounts of nebulised isoproterenol in status asthmaticus. *J. Allergy*, **43**, 101–13
32. van Schayck, C. P., Dompeling, E., van Herwaarden, C. L. A., Folgering, H., Verbeek, A. L. M., van der Hoogen, H. J. M. and van Weel, C. (1991). Bronchodilator treatment in moderate asthma or chronic bronchitis: continuous or on demand? A randomised controlled study. *Br. Med. J.*, **303**, 1426–31
33. O'Donnell, T. V. (1988). Asthma – Australia and New Zealand. *Aust. N. Z. J. Med.*, **18**, 303–10

DISCUSSION

Prof. P. Burney (London) With regard to the other aspect mentioned only briefly, the small gradual increase, it seems from the New Zealand data – and some rather more indirect information from the UK – that this gradual increase may well have started early in the century, in the 1920s or 1930s. From other evidence, the general prevalence of atopic disease in general also seems to be increasing, for instance, the prevalence of eczema. It is always difficult to evaluate historical data as well as current data, but do you not think that perhaps these other issues ought also to be considered, and that we should not look specifically at just one hypothesis to explain everything?

Dr R. Beasley I agree. One of my concerns is that some people are proposing that this gradual increase may relate solely to the regular use of β-agonist drugs. As you mentioned, particularly looking at the New Zealand experience, the increase actually began in the 1940s to 1950s. A similar increase has now been identified from the experience in Australia and the UK. I think we should concentrate not only on pharmacological changes but also on the non-pharmacological changes that have occurred during this period, in particular whether this gradual increase in mortality may relate to increased exposure to allergens or changes in the way in which this exposure is handled. These are just as feasible hypotheses, if not more so.

Dr J. Costello (London) The fact that the van Schayck study also implicated anticholinergics will also be significant.

Dr R. Beasley Yes. The van Schayck study suggests that adverse long-term effects may occur with the regular use of other bronchodilator drugs such as anticholinergics, as well as β-agonist drugs. Their findings also provide support for the view that inhaled β-agonists should be used on an 'as required' basis, rather than according to a regular scheduled regimen.

9

β-Agonist-induced hyper-responsiveness of the airways

A. E. Tattersfield

This chapter will discuss the evidence that β-agonists can increase airway responsiveness, the possible mechanisms underlying such an increase and its clinical significance. Before discussing any increase in airway responsiveness with β-agonists it is important to recognize that β-agonists when given acutely will cause the opposite effect, a reduction in airway responsiveness. Whether β-agonists reduce or increase bronchial responsiveness depends on the duration of treatment and, more crucially, on the time after inhalation when the response is measured.

ACUTE EFFECTS

Single doses of β_2-agonists provide protection against all constrictor stimuli in subjects with asthma including exercise, allergen, histamine and methacholine; the degree of protection is related to the dose of β-agonist administered[1]. This non-specific protective effect is analogous to the functional antagonism seen *in vitro* where β_2-agonists cause airway relaxation irrespective of the constrictor stimulus[2–5]. β-Agonists may alter airway calibre through other mechanisms however, including inhibition of mediator release from inflammatory cells in the lung[6–11], reduction of parasympathetic discharge from cholinergic ganglia[12,13], an increase in the volume and viscosity of mucus or through a reduction in vascular permeability and oedema in the airways.

In single-dose studies in asthmatic subjects, inhaled β_2-agonists reduce the provocative dose of histamine or methacholine which causes a 20% fall in forced expiratory volume (FEV_1) (PD_{20}). The maximum reduction is usually of the order of two to four doubling doses of the constrictor agonists, i.e. four to sixteen times more histamine or methacholine can be given before the FEV_1 falls by 20%[1]. The time course of change in bronchial responsiveness is roughly similar to the time course of change in measures of bronchodilatation such as the FEV_1[14]. This is shown diagrammatically in Figure 1. Small doses of β_2-agonists inhibit the constrictor response to exercise[15] and the early response to antigen[16]; the late response to antigen is inhibited by high doses of salbutamol[17] and by the long-acting β_2-agonist salmeterol[18].

EFFECT OF REGULAR TREATMENT

The concern of this chapter is whether following regular administration of β_2-agonists there is a reduction in the protection afforded by β_2-agonists against constrictor stimuli and whether, after stopping treatment, there is a rebound increase in bronchial reactivity. These are shown diagrammatically in Figure 2.

Loss of protection against constrictor stimuli

In a study of oral salbutamol, 16 mg daily for between 4 and 20 weeks, Gibson and colleagues[19] found a reduction in the protective effect of inhaled salbutamol (200 μg) against an exercise challenge in asthmatic subjects although the bronchodilator response was maintained. There was a similar but non-significant trend in subjects receiving regular inhaled salbutamol (800 μg daily). After 2 weeks of regular treatment with inhaled terbutaline the protection provided by terbutaline against histamine-induced bronchoconstriction was reduced in subjects with mild asthma studied by Vathenen and colleagues[20]. A non-significant trend in the same direction has been seen in other studies[21,22].

Rebound increase in bronchial responsiveness

Six studies to date have shown a significant rebound increase in bronchial reactivity to histamine and methacholine in asthmatic subjects following treatment with regular β_2-agonists[20,22–26]. The increase in reactivity has occurred after fenoterol, salbutamol and terbutaline following treatment for periods ranging from 2 weeks to 52 weeks. The fall in PD_{20} has ranged from 0.6 to 1.7 doubling doses of histamine or methacholine. Other studies have failed to show significant changes[27–30] though the trend in almost all has been

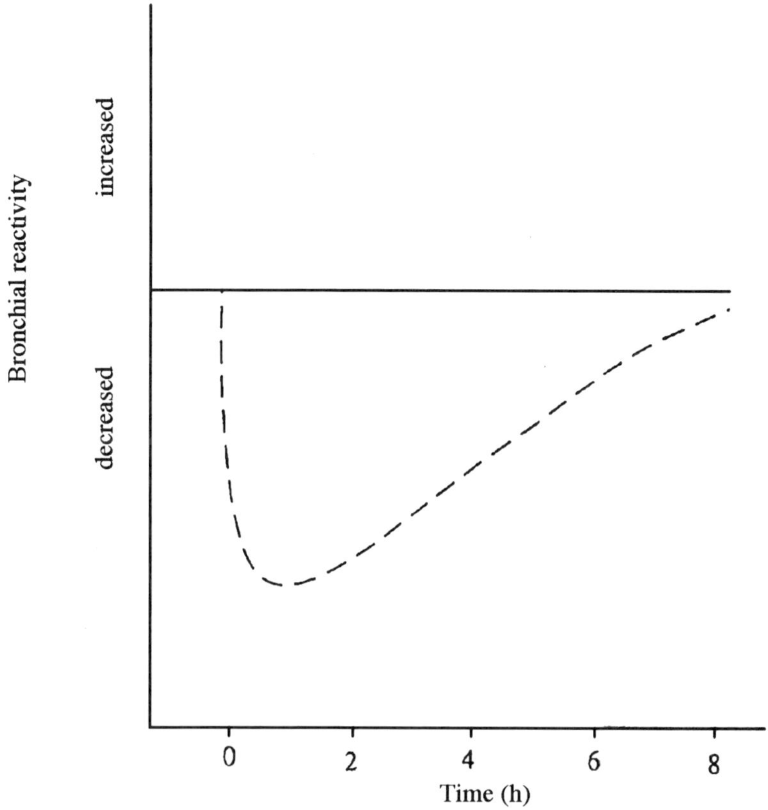

Figure 1 Diagrammatic representation of change in airway responsiveness to histamine or methacholine over 6 h of treatment. Following acute administration of a β-agonist there is a reduction in airway reactivity which has roughly the same time course as the bronchodilator response

towards an increase in bronchial reactivity (see Table 1; studies looking at changes at 6 h or less[31] or where there is no measurement prior to starting β-agonists[32] have not been included).

Certain conclusions can be drawn from the table. There is a clear trend towards an increased responsiveness overall following regular β_2-agonist treatment (the null hypothesis would be that a similar number of studies would show a significant decrease as show an increase in reactivity). This view is strengthened by the fact that the placebo-controlled studies have

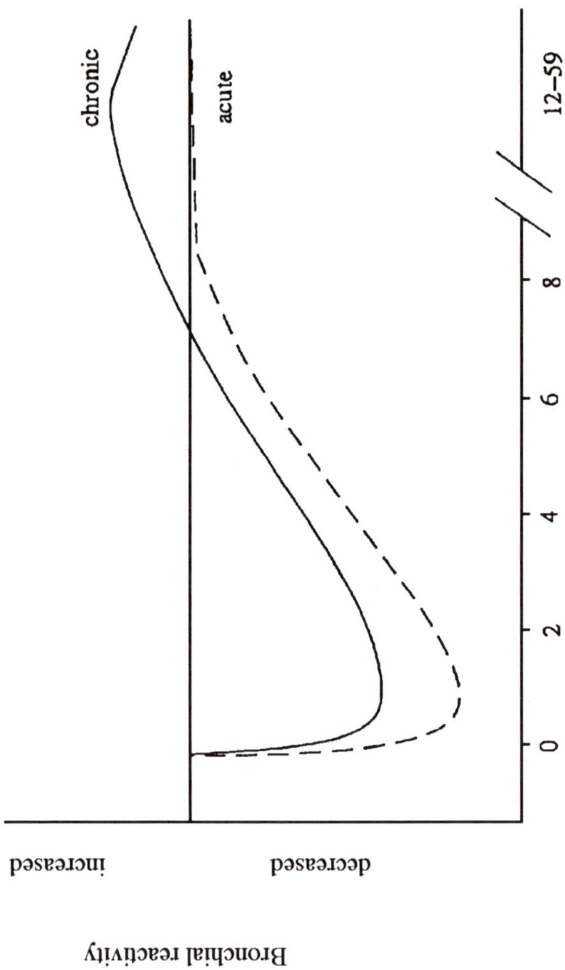

Figure 2 The question at issue is whether following regular treatment there is reduced protection by β-agonists against constrictor stimuli and/or a rebound increase in bronchial reactivity as shown by the solid line

Table 1 Change in provocative concentration (PC_{20}) or provocative dose (PD_{20}) required to reduce forced expiratory volume by 20% following cessation of regular treatment with β-agonists

	n	*Drug and dose*†	*Duration* (weeks)	*Interval after stopping* (hours)	*PD_{20} (or PC_{20}) in doubling doses* *(95% CI when given)*
Placebo-controlled studies					
Vathenen *et al.*[20]	8	terbutaline 750 μg t.d.s.	2	up to 23 h	– 1.5 (0.6–2.5)*
Wahedna *et al.*[22]	11	salbutamol 200 μg t.d.s.	3	up to 59 h	– 1.47 (0.6–2.4)*
		broxaterol 400 μg t.d.s.			– 0.95 (0.05–1.8)*
Sears *et al.*[26]	64	fenoterol 400 μg t.d.s.	24	> 6 h	– 0.6
Non-placebo-controlled studies					
Harvey and Tattersfield[28]	8	salbutamol up to 500 μg q.i.d.	4	12 h	
Peel and Gibson[27]	8	salbutamol 200 μg q.i.d.	4	> 6 h	– 0.25 NS
Kraan *et al.*[23]	17	terbutaline	2	12–16 h	– 0.8*
		500 μg q.i.d.	4		– 0.5 NS
Kerrebijn *et al.*[24]	7	terbutaline	4	12 h	– 0.9*
		200 μg t.d.s.	12		– 0.8*
			24		– 0.8*
Raes et al. 1989[29]	8	fenoterol 200 μg q.i.d.	16	about 12 h	+ 1.0
van Schayck *et al.*[25]	15	salbutamol	12	8–12 h	– 0.4*
		400 μg q.i.d.	24		– 0.7
van Schayck *et al.*[30]	21	salbutamol 400 μg q.i.d.	104	at least 8 h	– 0.5 NS

*Changes significant; NS, not significant; †t.d.s., three times daily; q.i.d., four times daily

shown a consistent increase. Second, the duration of treatment is not clearly related to the magnitude of the increase in airway responsiveness. Third, the magnitude of the increase in reactivity is in general larger in the studies which have a longer time interval between the last dose of β-agonist and the constrictor challenge. The time after cessation of treatment when the greatest change in bronchial reactivity occurs is still not clear however. In the study by Vathenen and colleagues[20] the greatest increase in bronchial responsiveness to histamine (1.5 doubling doses) was seen 23 h after cessation of treatment, the final time of measurement. In a more recent study, Wahedna and colleagues[22] continued to measure histamine responsiveness for up to 59 h after stopping regular salbutamol and found the greatest increase in bronchial reactivity (1.7 doubling doses) at this time. In this study the increase in bronchial responsiveness was associated with a 10% fall in FEV_1 and a fall has been seen in two other studies[25,26]. Most studies have looked at the effect of β-agonists on histamine or methacholine responsiveness since these are easier to study. One uncontrolled study showed an increased response to inhaled antigen in three patients following treatment[33] with a β-agonist but we have been unable to confirm this in a placebo-controlled study (C. Wong *et al.*, unpublished results).

MECHANISM UNDERLYING THE INCREASED REACTIVITY FOLLOWING β-AGONISTS

The mechanism underlying this rebound increase in bronchial responsiveness following β-agonist treatment has not been clarified. Possible mechanisms include:

(1) Desensitization of β-receptors on airway smooth muscle of inflammatory cells;

(2) Increased antigen deposition with β-agonist treatment causing an increase in bronchial responsiveness as occurs after an antigen challenge;

(3) Increased mucus production;

(4) Inhibition of mast cell release of heparin which has anti-inflammatory properties;

(5) Formulation of fenoterol as a bromide; and

(6) Effect of dextroisomers of β-agonists.

β-receptor desensitization

Regular administration of β-agonists causes a rapid and marked reduction in β-receptor numbers and function in human white cells *ex vivo*[34] and incubation with isoprenaline *in vitro* causes clear-cut desensitization to β-agonists in human airway smooth muscle[35,36]. Recent work has started to unravel the mechanisms underlying this desensitization[37–39]. Studies of tolerance to β-agonists in man have been less clear-cut. There is good evidence in both asthmatic and non-asthmatic subjects that tolerance occurs to non-airway responses following regular β_2-agonist treatment, including heart rate and tremor[40–43]. The main argument against β-receptor desensitization is that it has been difficult in general to demonstrate tolerance to the bronchodilating effects of β-agonists in patients with asthma[28,40,43]. One hypothesis which would explain most of the findings would be down-regulation of β-receptors on inflammatory cells following regular treatment with β-agonists. This would mean that when β-agonists were stopped, the inhibitory effect of circulating catecholamines on mediator release would be reduced; the consequent increase in mediator release might then increase bronchial reactivity. The loss of protection by β-agonists against constrictor challenge seen in some studies is more likely to relate to β-receptor down-regulation on airway smooth muscle.

Increased antigen deposition

It has been suggested that β-agonists, by causing bronchodilatation, might increase the amount of antigen inhaled and this would increase airway responsiveness[26,44]. Deposition of antigen would be expected to relate to minute volume more than airway calibre. β-agonists can increase minute volume[45] but the increase is very small in relation to the increase seen with exercise, for example. Since exercise has not caused a late increase in bronchial reactivity in most studies it seems unlikely that β-agonists would do so by this mechanism. Furthermore, if asthma improved with the β-agonist, minute ventilation would be expected to fall.

Increased production of mucus

Increased mucus production has been demonstrated *in vitro*[46] and has been noticed *in vivo* by normal subjects inhaling large doses of β-agonists during experiments (personal observation). It is perhaps unlikely that an increase in mucus would increase bronchial responsiveness but such a hypothesis is difficult to disprove.

Inhibition of mast cell release of heparin and other proteoglycans

By inhibiting mast cell mediator release, β-agonists inhibit the release of heparin and other proteoglycans which have anti-inflammatory activity in addition to inhibiting pro-inflammatory mediators, and it has been suggested that β-agonists could thereby increase airway inflammation[47] (see Chapter 3). If this mechanism was important β_2-agonists and other mast cell stabilizing drugs would be expected to increase inflammation in the airways. There are no data to support this as yet in man.

Formulation of fenoterol as a bromide

Since eosinophils oxidize bromide in preference to chloride, and bromide oxidants are capable of damaging cells[48] it was suggested that this might have been the mechanism underlying problems with fenoterol, which is formulated as a bromide[49,50]. This could not explain the increase in reactivity which has been seen with the other β-agonists which are not formulated as a bromide however.

Effect of dextro isomers of β-agonists

Work in guinea-pigs has suggested that the D-enantiomers of salbutamol and isoprenaline, which have no bronchodilating activity, may increase bronchial reactivity[44]. The authors suggest that the bronchodilator response to racemic salbutamol may not last as long as the adverse effects of D-salbutamol. Such effects have not been studied in man.

CLINICAL SIGNIFICANCE OF THE CHANGE IN BRONCHIAL RESPONSIVENESS

Although not all studies have produced a statistically significant increase in bronchial responsiveness following β_2-agonists the trend overall provides convincing evidence of a small increase in bronchial responsiveness following cessation of treatment with β-agonists. The regular use of β_2-agonists for as short a period as 2 weeks causes a rebound increase in bronchial reactivity several hours after cessation of treatment which continues for the following 2 to 3 days (Figure 2). An increase in bronchial responsiveness presumably means that patients would be more vulnerable to constrictor stimuli such as exercise or allergen. Although the mean changes are fairly small any increase in bronchial responsiveness could be important in a small proportion of patients with more severe hyper-responsiveness, and could conceivably cause a severe or even fatal attack of asthma on rare occasions. The fall in FEV_1 that was seen in two of the three placebo-controlled studies is in keeping with this. These changes would only be expected to be important if patients stopped taking their β-agonist and the magnitude of the effect may depend on other treatment they are taking such as inhaled steroids. In public health terms the evidence in the United Kingdom suggests that serious adverse effects from β_2-agonists must be rare or counterbalanced by beneficial effects since the threefold increase in β_2-agonist usage over the last decade has not been associated with any increase in asthma mortality.

ACKNOWLEDGEMENT

Some of the work has been reviewed in more detail in a chapter written with Dr Colin Wong and I acknowledge his help (in Beasley, R. (ed.), *Asthma Mortality*, CRC Press, Wellington, New Zealand).

REFERENCES

1. Tattersfield, A. E. (1987). Effect of beta-agonists and anticholinergic drugs on bronchial reactivity. *Am. Rev. Respir. Dis.*, **136**, S64–8
2. Mathe, A, A., Astrom, A. and Persson, N.-A. (1971). Some bronchoconstriction and bronchodilating responses of human isolated bronchi: evidence for the existence of alpha-adrenoceptors. *J. Pharm. Pharmacol.*, **23**, 905–10

3. Davis, C., Conolly, M. E. and Greenacre, J. K. (1980). Beta-adrenoceptors in human lung, bronchus and lymphocytes. *Br. J. Clin. Pharmacol.*, **10**, 425–32
4. Goldie, R. G., Spina, D., Henry, P. J., Lulich, K. M. and Paterson, J. W. (1986). *In vitro* responsiveness of human asthmatic bronchus to carbachol, histamine, beta-adrenoceptor agonists and theophylline. *Br. J. Clin. Pharmacol.*, **22**, 669–76
5. van Koppen, C. H., Rodrigues de Miranda, J. F., Beld, A. J. and van Ginneken, C. A. M. (1989). β-adrenoceptor binding and induced relaxation in airway smooth muscle from patients with chronic airflow obstruction. *Thorax*, **44**, 28–35
6. Assem, E. S. K. and Schild, H. O. (1969). Inhibition by sympathomimetic amines of histamine release induced by antigen in passively sensitized human lung. *Nature (London)*, **224**, 1028–9
7. Butchers, P. R., Fullarton, J. R., Skidmore, I. F., Thompson, L. E., Vardey, C. J. and Wheeldon, A. (1979). A comparison of the anti-anaphylactic activities of salbutamol and disodium cromoglycate in the rat, the rat mast cell and in human lung tissue. *Br. J. Pharmacol.*, **67**, 23–32
8. Radermecker, M. and Guston, M. (1981). An *in vivo* demonstration of the anti-anaphylactic effect of terbutaline. *Clin. Allergy*, **11**, 79–86
9. Marone, G., Kagey-Sobotka, A. and Lichtenstein, L. M. (1979). Effects of arachidonic acid and its metabolites on antigen-induced histamine release from human basophils *in vitro*. *J. Immunol.*, **123**, 1669–77
10. Peters, S P., Schulman, E. S., Schleimer, R. P., Macglashan, D. W., Newball, H. H. and Lichtenstein, L. M. (1982). Dispersed human lung mast cells. Pharmacological aspects and comparison with human lung tissue fragments. *Am. Rev. Respir. Dis.*, **126**, 1034–9
11. Butchers, P. R., Skidmore, I. F., Vardey, C. J. and Wheeldon, A. (1980). Characterization of the receptor mediating the anti-anaphylactic effects of beta-adrenoceptor agonists in human lung tissue *in vitro*. *Br. J. Pharmacol.*, **71**, 663–7
12. Skoogh, B. E. (1983). Transmission through airway ganglia. *Eur. J. Respir. Dis.*, **64** (Suppl. 131), 159–70
13. Rhoden, K. J., Meldrum, L. A. and Barnes, P. J. (1988). Inhibition of cholinergic neurotransmission in human airways by β_2-adrenoceptors. *J. Appl. Physiol.*, **65**, 700–5
14. Ahrens, R C., Harris, J. B., Milavetz, G., Annis, L. and Ries, R. (1987). Use of bronchial provocation with histamine to compare the pharmacodynamics

of inhaled albuterol and metaproterenol in patients with asthma. *J. Allergy Clin. Immunol.*, **79**, 876–82

15. Anderson, S. D., Seale, J. P., Rozea, P., Bandler, L., Theobald, G. and Lindsay, D. A. (1976). Inhaled and oral salbutamol in exercise induced asthma. *Am. Rev. Respir. Dis.*, **114**, 493–500
16. Cockcroft, D. W. and Murdock, K. Y. (1987). Comparative effects of inhaled salbutamol, sodium cromoglycate and beclomethasone dipropionate on allergen-induced early asthmatic responses, late asthmatic responses and increased bronchial responsiveness to histamine. *J. Allergy Clin. Immunol.*, **79**, 734–40
17. Twentyman, O. P., Finnerty, J. P. and Holgate, S. T. (1991). The inhibitory effects of nebulized albuterol on the early and late asthmatic reactions and increase in airway responsiveness provoked by inhaled allergen in asthma. *Am. Rev. Respir. Dis.*, **144**, 782–7
18. Twentyman, O. P., Finnerty, J. P., Harris, A., Palmer, J. and Holgate, S. T. (1990). Protection against allergen-induced asthma in salmeterol. *Lancet*, **336**, 1338–42
19. Gibson, G. J., Greenacre, J. K., Konig, P., Conolly, M. E. and Pride, N. B. (1978). Use of exercise challenge to investigate possible tolerance to beta-adrenoceptor stimulation in asthma. *Br. J. Dis. Chest*, **72**, 199–206
20. Vathenen, A. S., Knox, A. J., Higgins, B. G., Britton, J. R. and Tattersfield, A. E. (1988). Rebound increase in bronchial responsiveness after treatment with inhaled terbutaline. *Lancet*, **1**, 554–8
21. Harvey, J. E., Baldwin, C. J., Wood, P. J., Alberti, K. G. M. M. and Tattersfield, A. E. (1981). Airway and metabolic responsiveness to intravenous salbutamol in asthma: effect of regular inhaled salbutamol. *Clin. Sci.*, **60**, 579–85
22. Wahedna, I., Wisniewski, A., Wong, C., Pavord, I. and Tattersfield, A. E. (1991). Airway effects of regular broxaterol and salbutamol treatment in asthmatic subjects. *Thorax*, **46**, 770P
23. Kraan, J., Koeter, G. H., van der Mark, T. H., Sluiter, H. J. and de Vries, K. (1985). Changes in bronchial reactivity induced by 4 weeks of treatment with anti-asthmatic drugs in patients with allergic asthma: a comparison between budesonide and terbutaline. *J. Allergy Clin. Immunol.*, **76**, 628–36
24. Kerrebijn, K. F., van Essen-Zandvliet, E. E. M. and Neijens, H. J. (1987). Effect of long term treatment with inhaled corticosteroids and beta agonists on the bronchial responsiveness in children with asthma. *J. Allergy Clin. Immunol.*, **79**, 653–9

25. van Schayck, C. P., Graafsma, S. J., Visch, M. B., Dompeling, E., van Weel, C. and van Herwaarden, C. L. A. (1990). Increased bronchial responsiveness after inhaling salbutamol during 1 year is not caused by subsensitization to salbutamol. *J. Allergy Clin. Immunol.*, **86**, 793–800
26. Sears, M. R., Taylor, D. R., Print, C. G., Lake, D. C., Li, Q., Flannery, E. M., Yates, D. M., Lucas, M. K. and Herbison, G. P. (1990). Regular inhaled beta-agonist treatment in bronchial asthma. *Lancet*, **336**, 1391–6
27. Peel, E. T. and Gibson, G. J. (1980). Effects of long-term inhaled salbutamol therapy on the provocation of asthma by histamine. *Am. Rev. Respir. Dis.*, **121**, 973–8
28. Harvey, J. E. and Tattersfield, A. E. (1982). Airway response to salbutamol: effect of regular salbutamol inhalations in normal, atopic, and asthmatic subjects. *Thorax*, **37**, 280–7
29. Raes, M., Mulder, P. and Kerrebijn, K. F. (1989). Long-term effect of ipratropium bromide and fenoterol on the bronchial hyperresponsiveness to histamine in children with asthma. *J. Allergy Clin. Immunol.*, **84**, 874–9
30. van Schayck, C. P., Dompeling, E., van Herwaarden, C. L. A., Folgerin, H., Verbeek, A. L. M. van der Hoogen, H. J. M. and van Weel, C. (1991). Bronchodilator treatment in moderate asthma or chronic bronchitis: continuous or on demand? A randomised controlled study. *Br. Med. J.*, **303**, 1426–31
31. Joad, J. P., Ahrens, R. C., Lindgren, S. D. and Weinberger, M. M. (1987). Relative efficacy of maintenance therapy with theophylline, inhaled albuterol, and the combination for chronic asthma. *J. Allergy Clin. Immunol.*, **79**, 78–85
32. Haahtela, T., Jarvinen, M., Kava, T., Kiviranta, K., Koskinen, S., Lehtonen, K., Nikander, K., Persson, T., Reinikainen, K., Selroos, O., Sovijarvi, A., Stenius-Aarniala, B., Svahn, T., Tammivaara, R. and Laitinen, L. A. (1991). Comparison of a beta$_2$-agonist, terbutaline, with an inhaled corticosteroid, budesonide, in newly detected asthma. *N. Engl. J. Med.*, **325**, 388–92
33. Tashkin, D. P., Conolly, M. E., Deutsch, R. I., Hui, K. K., Littner, M., Scarpace, P. and Abrass, I. (1982). Subsensitization of beta-adrenoceptors in airways and lymphocytes of healthy and asthmatic subjects. *Am. Rev. Respir. Dis.*, **125**, 185–93
34. Galant, S. P., Duriseti, L., Underwood, S. and Insel, P. A. (1978). Decreased beta-adrenergic receptors on polymorphonuclear leukocytes after adrenergic therapy. *N. Engl. J. Med.*, **299**, 933–6
35. Davis, C. and Conolly, M. E. (1980). Tachyphylaxis to beta-adrenoceptor agonists in human bronchial smooth muscle: studies *in vitro*. *Br. J. Clin. Pharmacol.*, **10**, 417–23

36. Avner, B. P. and Jenne, J. W. (1981). Desensitisation of isolated human bronchial smooth muscle to beta-receptor agonists. *J. Allergy Clin. Immunol.*, **68**, 51–7
37. Sibley, D. R. and Lefkowitz, R. J. (1985). Molecular mechanisms of receptor desensitisation using the beta-adrenergic receptor-coupled adenylate cyclase system as a model. *Nature (London)*, **317**, 124–9
38. Lefkowitz, R. J., Hausdorff, W. P. and Caron, M. G. (1990). Role of phosphorylation in desensitization of the β-adrenoceptor. *Trends Pharmacol. Sci.*, **11**, 190–4
39. Hausdorf, W. P., Caron, M. G. and Lefkowitz, R. J. (1990). Turning off the signal: desensitisation of beta-adrenergic receptor function. *FASEB J.*, **4**, 2881–9
40. Larsson, S., Svedmyr, N. and Thiringer, G. (1977). Lack of bronchial beta-adrenoceptor resistance in asthmatics during long-term treatment with terbutaline. *J. Allergy Clin. Immunol.*, **59**, 93–100
41. Lipworth, B. J., Struthers, A. D. and McDevitt, D. G. (1989). Tachyphylaxis to systemic but not to airway responses during prolonged therapy with high dose inhaled salbutamol in asthmatics. *Am. Rev. Respir. Dis.*, **140**, 586–92
42. Holgate, S. T., Stubbs, W. A., Wood, P. J., McCaughey, E. S., Alberti, K. G. M. M. and Tattersfield, A. E. (1980). Airway and metabolic resistance to intravenous salbutamol: a study in normal man. *Clin. Sci.*, **59**, 155–61
43. Tattersfield, A. E. (1985). Tolerance to beta agonists. *Bull. Eur. Physiopathol. Respir. (Clin. Respir. Physiol.)*, **21**, 1–5s
44. Morley, J., Sanjar, S. and Newth, C. (1990). Viewpoint: untoward effects of beta-adrenoceptor agonists in asthma. *Eur. Respir. J.*, **3**, 228–33
45. Rudolf, M., Turner, J., Summers, G., Ullah, M., Good, C. and Stanley, N. (1979). Effect of beta-adrenergic blockade and stimulation on respiration. *Thorax*, **34**, 701–2
46. Borson, B. and Nadel, J. (1986). Neurophysiologic control of airway secretions in experimental animals. *Am. Rev. Respir. Dis.*, **134**, 614–17
47. Page, C. P. (1991). Hypothesis: one explanation of the asthma paradox: inhibition of natural anti-inflammatory mechanism by beta$_2$-agonists. *Lancet*, **337**, 717–20
48. Slungaard, A. and Mahoney, J. R. (1991). Bromide-dependent toxicity of eosinophil peroxidase for endothelium and isolated working rat hearts: a model for eosinophilic endocarditis. *J. Exp. Med.*, **173**, 117–26
49. Green, W. F. (1991). Fenoterol and its bromide. *Lancet*, **337**, 1613

50. Hammer, R., Jennewein, H.-M., Kutter, E. and Lopez-Vidriero, M. T. (1991). Fenoterol and its bromide. *Lancet*, **338**, 507

DISCUSSION

Dr J. Costello (London) No differences seem to have been observed in patients who were using high doses of nebulized drugs – no dose-related phenomenon, for instance, either for withdrawal or increased hyper-reactivity, in comparison to the huge increase in the amount of nebulized drug that is certainly being used in this country?

Prof. A. E. Tattersfield A lot of the nebulized drugs are being used in older patients. The mortality data I discussed were in the younger group. With regard to reduction of the use of β-agonists, my own view is that proper trials of their reduction have to be done under controlled conditions. Such trials are quite difficult to do, but it seems to me, that is the only way to be able to answer these questions. As subtle an effect as that described by Dr Sears could be happening, and is difficult to exclude without doing proper studies.

Dr J. Morley (Basle, Switzerland) Your suggestion that desensitization of inflammatory cells might cause some adverse effect is, I suggest, at variance with observations in the guinea-pig – a classical animal for looking at this sort of situation. As we and many others before us have shown, it is clear that if high doses of sympathomimetics are given over a period of time the animals become very susceptible to either spasmogens or allergen (which is the situation here). We showed – and I think it is important – that in this situation the animals can very easily be protected simply by giving them either inhaled (which is particularly effective) or even systemic sympathomimetic therapy.

I think the cells are still capable of being protected, and I do not think your explanation fits the facts as seen in that classical model situation.

Prof. A. E. Tattersfield I was trying to explain the findings in man, which obviously are relevant, in that there is still this responsiveness to β-agonists when inhaled, yet there is the rebound increase in reactivity, and we can show that circulating cells will desensitize very easily.

10

Is there a place for long-acting β-agonists in asthma therapy?

R. W. Fuller

INTRODUCTION

The role of β_2-agonists in the treatment of asthma has again come under scrutiny. This follows a second increase in asthma deaths during the 1980s which has been associated with β_2-agonist use[1]. In addition, some studies have suggested that the regular use of β_2-agonists may be associated with a reduced control of asthma[2]. The newly available long-acting β_2-agonist salmeterol has led to the questioning of the place of β_2-agonists in asthma management[3]. To obtain maximum benefit from the long-acting drug it needs to be used as a prophylactic rather than as a symptomatic therapy as it is under these circumstances that the 12-h duration of action gives it advantage over the shorter acting drugs. Thus, if the various concerns over the use of β_2-agonists were to be substantiated then its role would be unclear. However, the evidence is not so clear cut and does not appear to be sufficient to deny use of salmeterol in clinical practice. This chapter will review the evidence on the effects of β_2-agonists in asthma from the literature and from that which is now available from the salmeterol programme.

EFFECT OF SHORT-ACTING β_2-AGONISTS

On mortality

Asthma is a potentially fatal disease and the mortality rate from asthma is not static. Analysis of the death rate in the UK over the last century has shown increases in the late 19th century, 1940s, 1960s and 1980s (Figure 1)[4]. The 'epidemic' in the 1960s was extensively studied in the UK and some other countries. There were a number of hypotheses which were widely discussed;

these included isoprenaline use, aerosol propellants, inadequate therapy and environmental effects. The matter was not resolved; however, the consensus did not come down against β_2-agonist use but in favour of an overall improvement in therapy[3].

The increase in deaths in the 1970s and 1980s in New Zealand has received equal attention and again β_2-agonist therapy was linked to the deaths[1]. Despite obvious associations with a number of different therapies, e.g. nebulized β_2-agonist and theophylline, and with severity, the association with fenoterol was the focus of most attention.

Recently, a survey of 44 asthma deaths in Saskatchewan, which is discussed in an earlier chapter by Spitzer, has also linked the asthma deaths to fenoterol, and for the first time to salbutamol use. However, salbutamol was not associated with an increase in overall mortality unlike fenoterol. Like the previous analysis of the association with death, the study was unable to dissociate drug use from severity of disease. It is certain that increased β_2-agonist use is most likely to occur in those patients with the worse disease and this will inevitably link the drug to asthma death.

Fortunately in the UK the death rate is now falling despite the increased use of β_2-agonists (Figure 1). Probably the important message from the analysis of death is the recognition by doctors that patients with increasing requirements for β_2-agonists require close assessment as they are likely to have severe disease.

On morbidity

β_2-Agonists in addition to being potent bronchodilators are effective as inhibitors of mediator release *in vitro*. This property has led to the study of their use as a potential disease modifying therapy. The regular use of short-acting β_2-agonists was shown in some patient groups to give sufficient protection against induced bronchospasm to reduce symptoms[3]. However, their regular use has not been shown to have clinically important effects on disease markers such as bronchial reactivity[3]. Bronchial reactivity during treatment with β_2-agonists has been the subject of a number of studies (Table 1) which have compared them to other therapies such as steroids as well as to placebo controls. The overall pattern showed neither an increase nor a reduction in bronchial reactivity.

More recently, two studies have suggested that regular therapy may be associated with poor asthma control[2] and a reduction in lung function over

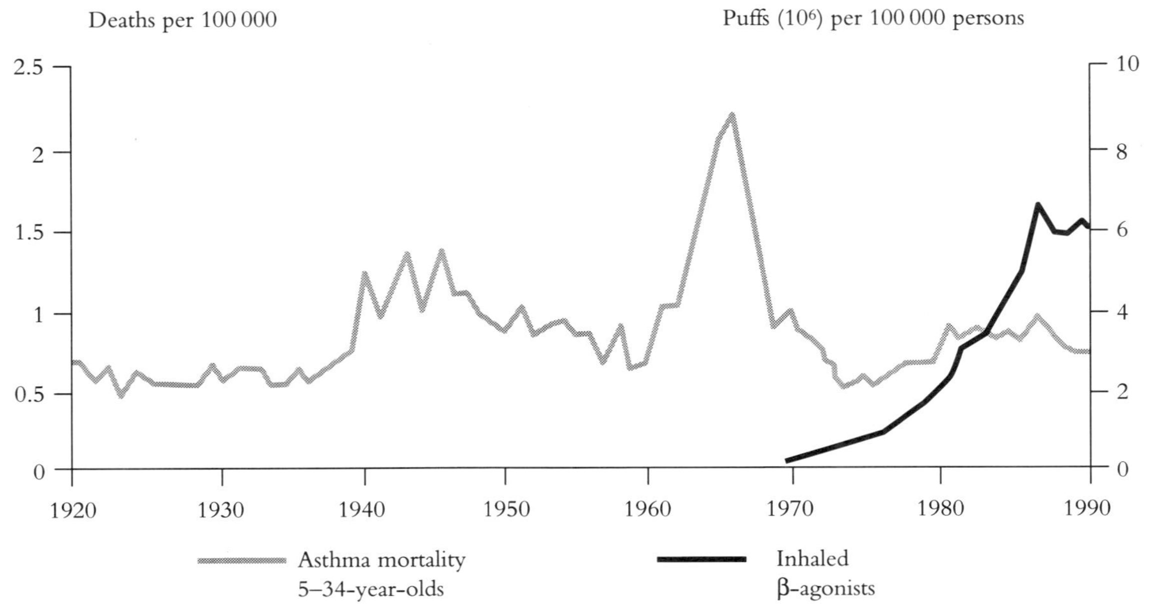

Figure 1 Asthma mortality in England and Wales compared to use of β_2-agonists in 5–34-year-olds between 1920 and 1990

Table 1 Bronchial reactivity during treatment with β_2-agonists measured as change in provocative concentration required to produce a 20% fall in forced expiratory volume (PC_{20})

Reference	*Authors*	*Number of patients*	*Months of treatment*	*Change in PC_{20}*
12	Bennati *et al.*	10	1	0.27
13	Haahtela *et al.*	53	24	0.5
14	Harvey and Tattersfield	8	1	NC
15	Joad *et al.*	18	1	< 1
16	Kerrebijn *et al.*	7	6	− 0.71
17	Kraan *et al.*	20	1	− 0.31
18	Peel and Gibson	8	1	− 0.19
19	Raes *et al.*	8	4	0.91
20	Vathenen *et al.*	8	0.5	↑
21	Van Schayck *et al.*	15	12	− 0.12
5	Van Schayck *et al.*	51	24	↑
22	Waalkens *et al.*	15	2	− 0.13
23	Woolcock *et al.*	11	24	− 0.12

NC = non-calculable; ↑ = increase

a 2-year period[5]. The study by Sears and colleagues has caused much interest and its individual analysis of the data does show a difference in the percentage of patients with better control, treated as required, compared to the regularly treated group. However, no data were presented to allow assessment of the magnitude of the effect. In addition, the recruitment requirements of patients entered into the study, which limited their severity, and the high drop-out rate, around 25%, make it difficult to assess its clinical relevance. Further independent analysis by the Committee on Safety of Medicines has suggested that the changes seen were small and of doubtful clinical relevance. The second study by Van Schayck and colleagues[5] made use of two drugs (salbutamol and ipratropium bromide) and was performed in a mixture of patients with chronic obstructive pulmonary disease and asthma. A greater decline in lung function was observed in patients treated regularly with both drugs compared to those treated as required with both drugs. However, there are clearly differences in the severity of the two patient populations and as anti-inflammatory therapy was stopped on entering into the study, it is conceivable that the deterioration on stopping this therapy was greater in the more severe patients, i.e. those treated with continuous therapy, questioning the clinical relevance of the study.

Table 2 Number of patients with asthma exacerbations during various time intervals comparing treatment with salbutamol (SAL) and beclomethasone (BDP) at different dosages

	Time interval (weeks)						
	1–3	*4–9*	*10–15*	*16–21*	*22–27*	*28–33*	*34–39*
Treatment: SAL 2000 μg q.i.d. + BDP 1000 μg b.i.d.							
Number of patients	51	47	43	41	37	35	32
Number of patients with one exacerbation	2	0	0	1	0	0	0
Treatment: SAL 2000 μg q.i.d. + BDP 500 μg b.i.d							
Number of patients	48	43	38	38	35	34	32
Number of patients with one exacerbation	2	1	0	0	0	1	0
Treatment: SAL 2000 μg q.i.d. + placebo							
Number of patients	49	42	39	33	29	26	19
Number of patients with one exacerbation	2	2	1	2	1	1	0
Total number of patients	148	132	120	112	101	95	83
Number of patients with one exacerbation	6	3	1	3	1	2	0

q.i.d., four times a day; b.i.d., twice a day

Data are available from the investigation of regular and conventional dose salbutamol from recent programmes within Glaxo. In one study over 9 months, 2 mg of salbutamol were taken four times a day, as sole therapy or in combination with beclomethasone. In this study there was neither an increase in exacerbation rate (Table 2) nor a decline in lung function, which is surprising if the adverse effects of β_2-agonists are dose-related. Treatment for 12 months of patients with salbutamol was not associated with any decline in lung function even in patients who were not receiving anti-inflammatory therapy[6], nor was there any increase in exacerbation rate over a 12-month period[7].

The case of β_2-agonists increasing asthma morbidity is therefore not proven. In fact, taken altogether, the data from various studies suggest that the short-acting β_2-agonist neither improved nor caused deterioration in asthma control.

SALMETEROL

Dose-finding studies

Single and multiple dose studies for up to 3 months have compared doses from 12.5 to 200 μg twice a day in both adults and children. In mild to moderate patients of all ages 50 mg twice a day is more effective than the lower doses[8] and salbutamol given four times a day[8]. This dose is not associated with any significant systemic effects[8]. In more severe asthmatics, especially those requiring oral prednisolone as maintenance therapy, 100 μg twice a day was more effective than 50 μg twice a day[9].

Long-term studies

The effect of salmeterol both from the metered dose inhaler and dry powder inhaler has been assessed in 3- and 12-month studies with both active (salbutamol)[10] and placebo controls. Salmeterol increases morning and evening peak flow, reduces symptoms and use of β_2-agonists for relief without any evidence of pharmacologically predictable side-effects in excess of those from the active comparator[10]. This effect of salmeterol is maintained throughout the 3-month studies where it has been intensively studied[10]. The effect of salmeterol was independent of the other therapy being used. In particular, in those patients not receiving concurrent anti-inflammatory therapy there was no loss of control over either 3 (Figure 2) or 12 months (Figure 3). The effect of salmeterol on use of β_2-agonists for relief was most marked in patients who required the greatest number of doses before randomization. Thus, regular salmeterol in these patients greatly reduced the total β-agonist load. If the use of salmeterol over a 12-month period were to be associated with loss of asthma control then this would be reflected with an increase of exacerbation rate. In neither of the two studies where salmeterol was given for 12 months was there any indication of such an effect[7]. If anything, there was a tendency for the exacerbation to fall (Figure 4).

The occurrence of death during the trials with salmeterol and its early use in clinical practice have been examined. The United Kingdom Committee on Safety of Medicines has reported 48 deaths (not all of them from asthma) during the first 6 months of its use. In isolation a high figure, however, an estimated death rate from the number of patients receiving salmeterol (> 400 000) would have been in excess of 100. This suggests that

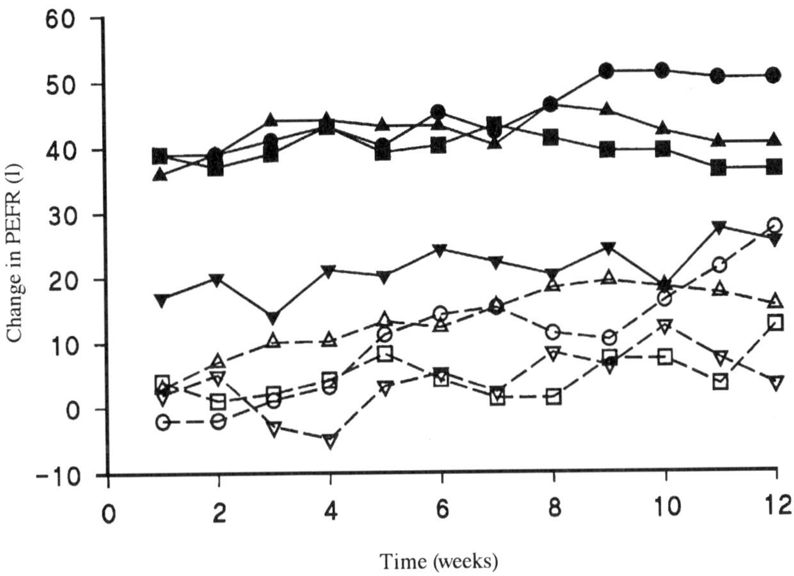

Figure 2 Change in morning peak expiratory flow rate (PEFR) on salbutamol (200 μg four times a day) and salmeterol (50 μg twice a day; solid symbols) over 3 months: ○, ●, no steroids; □, ■,< 1 mg, inhaled; △, ▲, > 1 mg, inhaled; ▽, ▼, oral therapy

despite its use in the most severe patients it was not associated with excess mortality.

Comparative studies

Previously, the oral route was the only one available for giving prolonged bronchodilatation. The use of both theophylline and sustained-release β_2-agonists is associated with a high incidence of systemic side-effects and they are therefore poorly tolerated by many patients. Salmeterol has proved to be more effective and better tolerated than titrated theophylline[11] and oral terbutaline. This is particularly evident in the control of nocturnal asthma and the overnight fall in peak flow, although day time symptoms and the use of rescue medication are also reduced.

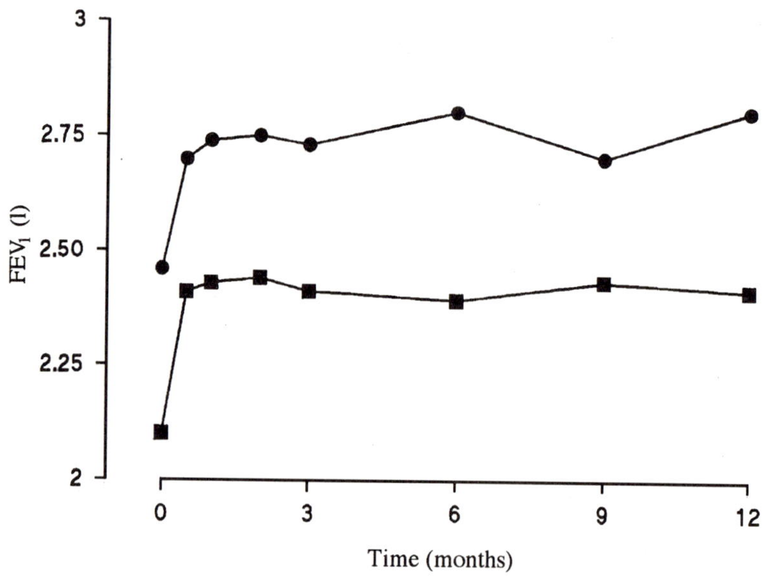

Figure 3 Forced expiratory volume at 1 second (FEV1) on salmeterol in two studies over 12 months: ●, dry powder TO6 (n = 175); ■, metered dose inhaler (n = 263)

Salmeterol has been compared to the putative anti-inflammatory agent sodium cromoglycate, and has proven to be a more effective agent at symptomatic relief and peak flow control in both adults and children. Thus, salmeterol appears to be a suitable replacement therapy for oral bronchodilators and the non-steroidal prophylactic agents. Its use is appropriate in patients requiring frequent doses of short-acting relief despite other appropriate therapy.

CONCLUSION

Despite close scrutiny and much debate the case that β_2-agonists increase asthma mortality and morbidity has not been proven. The use of salmeterol in large scale (> 6000) patient clinical studies and closely observed use in clinical practice do not reveal any evidence of deterioration of asthma control or increase in severe exacerbations or death during this therapy.

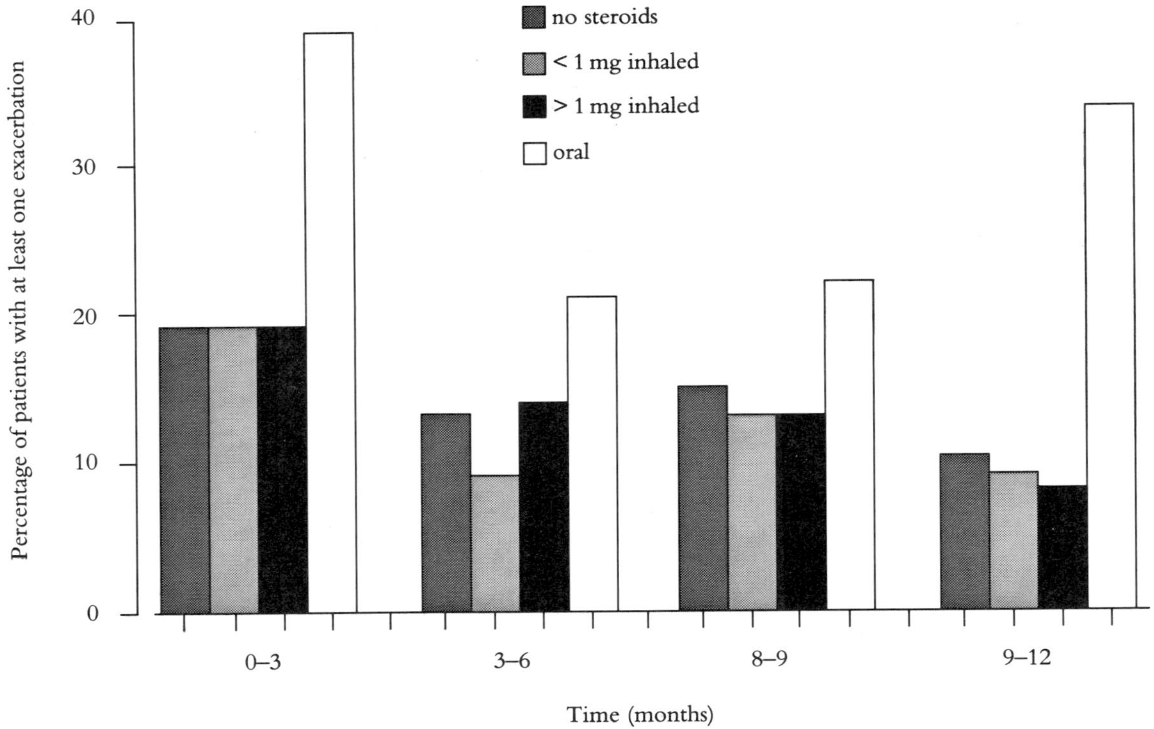

Figure 4 Asthma exacerbations according to steroid use: % of patients with at least one exacerbation on salmeterol, 50 μg twice a day is shown against time

Salmeterol is a safe and effective alternative to multiple doses of short-acting β_2-agonists as well as to oral bronchodilators and non-steroidal asthma prophylatic agents.

REFERENCES

1. Pearce, N., Crane, J., Burgess, C., Jackson, R. and Beasley, R. (1991). Beta agonists and asthma mortality: déjà vu. *Clin. Exp. Allergy*, **21**, 401–10
2. Sears, M. R., Taylor, D. R., Print, C. G., Lake, D. C., Li, Q., Flannery, E. M., Yates, D. M., Lucas, M. K. and Herbison, G. P. (1990). Regular inhaled beta-agonist treatment in bronchial asthma. *Lancet*, **336**, 1391–6
3. Lofdahl, C. G. and Svedmyr, N. (1991). Beta-agonists – friends or foes? *Eur. Respir. J.*, **4**, 1161–5
4. Speizer, F. E. and Doll, R. (1968). A century of asthma deaths in young people. *Br. Med. J.*, **3**, 245–6
5. Van Schayck, C. P., Dompeling, E., Van Herwaarden, C. L. A., Folgering, H., Verbeek, A. L. M., Van Der Hoogen, H. J. M. and Van Weel, C. (1991). Bronchodilator treatment in moderate asthma or chronic bronchitis: continuous or on demand? A randomised controlled study. *Br. Med. J.*, **303**, 1426–31
6. Fuller, R. W. and Hilton, C. J. (1992). Bronchodilator treatment in asthma: continuous or on demand? *Br. Med. J.*, **304**, 121
7. Shepherd, G. L., Jenkins, W. J. and Alexander, J. (1991). Asthma exacerbations in patients taking regular salmeterol or salbutamol for symptoms. *Lancet*, **337**, 1424
8. Dahl, R., Earnshaw, J. S. and Palmer, J. B. D. (1991). Salmeterol: a four week study of a long-acting beta-adrenoceptor agonist for the treatment of reversible airways disease. *Eur. Respir. J.*, **4**, 1178–84
9. Faurschou, P. (1991). Chronic dose-ranging studies with salmeterol. *Eur. Respir. Rev.*, **4**, 282–7
10. Britton, M. (1991). Salmeterol and salbutamol: large multicentre studies. *Eur. Respir. Rev.*, **4**, 288–92
11. Palmer, J. B. D. (1991). Salmeterol in clinical practice. *Eur. Respir. Rev.*, **4**, 297–300
12. Bennati, D., Piacentini, G. L., Peroni, G., Sette, L., Testi, R. and Boner, A. L. (1989). Changes in bronchial reactivity in asthmatic children after treatment with beclomethasone alone or in association with salbutamol. *J. Asthma*, **26**, 359–64

13. Haahtela, T., Jarvinen, M., Kavam T., Kiranta, K., Koskinen, S., Lehtonen, K., Nikander, K., Persson, T., Reinikainen, K., Selrdon, O., Sovjarvi, A., Steind-Aarniala, B. S., Svarn, T., Tammivaara, R. and Laitinen, L. A. (1991). Comparison of a β_2-agonist, terbutaline with an inhaled corticosteroid, budesonide in newly detected asthma. *N. Engl. J. Med.*, **325**, 388–92
14. Harvey, J. E. and Tattersfield, A. E. (1982). Airway response to salbutamol: effect of regular salbutamol inhalations in normal, atopic and asthmatic subjects. *Thorax*, **37**, 280–7
15. Joad, J. P., Ahrens, R. C., Lindgren, S. D. and Weinberger, M. M. (1987). Relative efficacy of maintenance therapy with theophylline, inhaled albuterol and the combination for chronic asthma. *J. Allergy Clin. Immunol.*, **79**, 78–85
16. Kerrebijn, K. F., van Essen-Zandvliet, E. E. M. and Neijens, H. J. (1987). Effect of long term treatment with inhaled corticosteroids and beta-agonists on the bronchial responsiveness in children with asthma. *J. Allergy Clin. Immunol.*, **79**, 653–9
17. Kraan, J., Koeter, G. H., van der Mark, T. W., Sluiter, H. J. and de Vries, K. (1985). Changes in bronchial hyperreactivity induced by 4 weeks of treatment with antiasthmatic drugs in patients with allergic asthma: a comparison between budesonide and terbutaline. *J. Allergy Clin. Immunol.*, **76**, 628–36
18. Peel, E. T. and Gibson, G. J. (1980). Effects of long-term inhaled salbutamol therapy on the provocation of asthma by histamine. *Am. Rev. Respir. Dis.*, **121**, 973–8
19. Raes, M., Mulder, P. and Kerrebijn, K. F. (1989). Long-term effect of ipratropium bromide and fenoterol on the bronchial hyperresponsiveness to histamine in children with asthma. *J. Allergy Clin. Immunol.*, **84**, 874–9
20. Vathenen, A. S., Knox, A. J., Higgins, B. G., Britton, J. R. and Tattersfield, A. E. (1988). Rebound increase in bronchial responsiveness after treatment with inhaled terbutaline. *Lancet*, **1**, 554–7
21. Van Schayck, C. P., Graafsma, S. J., Visch, M. B., Dompeling, E., van Weel, C. and van Herwaarden, C. L. A. (1990). Increased bronchial hyperresponsiveness after inhaling salbutamol during 1 year is not caused by subsensitization to salbutamol. *J. Allergy Clin. Immunol.*, **86**, 793–800
22. Waalkens, H. J., Gerritsen, J., Koeter, G. H., Krouwels, F. H., van Aalderen, W. M. C. and Knol, K. (1991). Budesonide and terbutaline or terbutaline alone in children with mild asthma: effects on bronchial hyperresponsiveness and diurnal variation in peak flow. *Thorax*, **46**, 499–503

23. Woolcock, A. J., Yan, K. and Salome, C. M. (1988). Effect of therapy on bronchial hyperresponsiveness in the long-term management of asthma. *Clin. Allergy*, **18**, 165–76

DISCUSSION

Dr C. Page (London) We heard this morning that this long-acting β-agonist has a long side-chain that buries itself in the receptor, or certainly in the membrane. If animals or people are dosed for 12 or 16 weeks with this compound, is there an accumulation in tissues? Most of your data on biological half-lives or pharmacokinetics were based on plasma levels. I would be very interested to know what happens in the tissues. I asked this question at the Food and Drug Administration, without getting a sensible answer.

Dr R. W. Fuller We have no idea in humans because lungs have never been removed to find out. [Dr Page: This shows why animal experiments have to be done] Yes, indeed – I am sure Dr Johnson will comment on guinea-pigs (which I cannot do).

Dr M. Johnson (UK) This is a very good question. In the development programme behind salmeterol this drug was given to animals not for a few weeks but for 2 years at maximum tolerated oral and inhaled doses. The tissue distribution and accumulation of the drug were measured during this time using radiolabelled material. The bottom-line answer, the same answer as given to the Food and Drug Administration a year ago, is that there is no accumulation.

Dr J. Morley (Basle, Switzerland) You suggested in the opening sentence that most of the meeting previously was an attack on β-agonists. I wondered whether you thought Dr Johnson was also attacking the product. He referred to the fact that you have here a racemic mixture. It is well-known that racemic mixtures have interactions in terms of metabolism, absorption and distribution. In the case of this particular substance, both enantiomers are active at the receptor site and may interact there. Would you not therefore think it sensible to take the two enantiomers and study them individually in man?

Dr R. W. Fuller I am not sure that I would use the emotive term 'sensible'. It would certainly be interesting and worth doing if enough of the purified enantiomers could be obtained to do toxicology. I suspect all that would be found would be that the less active enantiomer has less effect on the airways.

There does not seem to be any problem with metabolism of this drug, in as much as once it gets out of the lung it is metabolized to inactive constituents and does not accumulate – as we have heard in animal studies – in the lung or outside. I am not sure what benefit there would necessarily be from doing these studies.

Round table discussion

Chairman: N. C. Barnes

Dr N. C. Barnes (London) I will concentrate first on the clinical studies because in many ways, as clinicians, we are interested in the result of these treatments.

First, this debate in some ways goes on in a rather silly fashion in that we behave as if the alternatives are *either* inhaled steroids *or* regular β_2-agonist use – which is clearly not the case. From our understanding, both of the pathology of asthma and of what is a disease-modifying agent, most people would now believe that in anything but the most trivial asthma the correct approach would be to start with inhaled corticosteroids. Therefore, what we are interested in, in terms of regular versus *pro re nata* β_2-agonists, is whether in those patients who are not adequately controlled on inhaled steroids it is both safe and appropriate to use regular β_2-agonists.

Secondly, as a class of compounds, β-agonists have stood the test of time. They have been used in respiratory medicine for a long time and clinicians have been happy with them. If we are going to throw out a therapy or change its use in a major way, we should ask for the same quality of data that as clinicians we would want to see for a new drug. This should be borne in mind very much in looking at these studies: that useful treatments are not thrown out on the basis of anecdotes when a new treatment would not be accepted solely on that basis.

I would like now to turn to Prof. Spitzer's study, which has not as yet been published (although it will be very soon). There are points for clarification in that study and probably other aspects of it in which the audience is interested.

First, Dr Howarth's comment about the nebulizers. It is clear, and clinicians have known for a number of years, that frequent β_2-agonist use is a marker of patients at risk of death and near-miss death from asthma. Is it a marker of severity or the cause of the problem? If it is just a marker of severity, the Saskatchewan study has simply reproduced what was already known. If, however, it is the cause of the problem, these are very new and important data.

The nebulizer data seem to me to differentiate this. By my calculation, the amount of nebulized treatment received if a nebulizer were taken regularly would be the equivalent of one canister of β_2-agonist per day. If the proposal is that the problem is due to the β_2-agonist itself rather than to inappropriate use by the patient, the death rate – or the odds ratio – for nebulized β_2-agonists would be expected to be very high. In fact, though, it was not really out of line with the other treatment. What is Dr Spitzer's comment on this?

Dr W. Spitzer (Montreal, Canada) First, that in the period of time in which the study was done the use of nebulizer was fairly infrequent in Saskatchewan (as borne out by the data from the prescription drug database). Whilst the odds ratios are lower than might have been expected on the basis of common sense, the confidence intervals are so wide that there may be some oscillation present that is nothing more than random error.

Secondly, some of the use of the product by nebulizer is in the context of a hospital event, which is not segregated separately in the prescription drug database. Not much store is set by that, therefore, and we did not hypothesize in advance because of that. There is frequent nebulizer use in hospitals in Saskatchewan that is not recorded in the prescription drug database, and so does not hit the numerator. This would not be the case for metered dose inhaler use.

Dr N. C. Barnes We are really interested in *home* treatment. Would your database pick up home nebulizer treatment? [Dr Spitzer assented] How may were on the home nebulizers, because that seems to me to be critical? The dose received by the nebulizer is so high that if it is a drug effect, [the odds ratio] would be expected to be very high.

Dr J. Moore-Gillon (London) Can you extract from your data information as to whether possession of a nebulizer is a marker for a patient under close medical supervision, whereas prescription of more than two inhalers a month is a marker for a patient who is not under close medical supervision?

Dr W. Spitzer This cannot be extracted from the computer data banks without doing a validation, which has not been done.

Dr M. Rudolf (Ealing) The other drugs that might be expected to be used more with increasing severity [of asthma] would be inhaled steroids, yet it was interesting that the odds ratio for inhaled steroids seemed to be very low. Is this because patients in Saskatchewan stop using their inhaled steroids as they become worse or do they use oral steroids instead?

Dr W. Spitzer The odds ratio for inhaled steroids was below 1 – and statistically significantly below 1 – which indicated a benefit, as opposed to a risk or harm. It was in the first part of the study period (which was from 1980 to 1987) that these drugs were introduced into the Saskatchewan formulary – in doses that might almost be called homeopathic. It is only when we get up to the use of 12 canisters per year (an average of one per month) that the conventional usual doses in Canada now – and presumably also in the UK and Europe – begin to be approached. Only when the way in which the product is used *now* is approached is the benefit seen as a clear low odds ratio below unity.
(Netherlands) Was ipratropium bromide also scored in the system and, if so, how does it relate to the β_2-agonists?

Dr W. Spitzer This drug was used relatively little. I cannot remember the numbers but, as I recall, it was not remarkably different from unity when taken separately, and it was not a prior hypothesis.

Dr R. Beasley (Wellington, New Zealand) When examining the class effect it is obviously very important that the controls on no inhaled β-agonist therapy have asthma of similar severity to the controls on inhaled β-agonist therapy. What evidence is there that they are of similar severity, and how many of the controls not on an inhaled β-agonist were in fact on no treatment at all during the 2-year study period? What effect is there on the analysis if any of those subjects are taken out of the subsequent analyses?

Dr W. Spitzer In my view, it would be inappropriate to take those subjects out of the analysis. Their experience is known; they do not exhibit characteristics as severe as those of the cases. Adjustment was made for these differences in the analysis in the way I described in logistic regression.

Dr N. C. Barnes That is a worry I have here. One would intuitively think that somebody who visits his doctor twice as often as somebody else probably does so because his asthma is rather worse. Are there any other data to indicate the matching of the groups – any peak flow data, for example, on these patients when they visited their physicians or were admitted to hospital?

Dr W. Spitzer There are data on approximately 40% of the subjects from field surveys in doctors' offices, hospitals and from records. As may be imagined, it is hard to get a good response rate going back up to 12 years in physicians', consultants' or general practitioners' records. We are concluding this analysis now – it is what I referred to as Part II of our work – and I am not ready to present it.

Index